IT'S NOT YOUR FAULT
IT'S YOUR HORMONES

Amazing New Diet Program for Women

MITCHELL R. SUSS

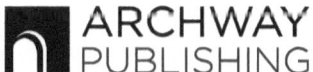
ARCHWAY
PUBLISHING

The information, ideas, and suggestions in this book are not intended as a substitute for professional medical advice. Before following any suggestions contained in this book, you should consult your personal physician. Neither the author nor the publisher shall be liable or responsible for any loss or damage allegedly arising as a consequence of your use or application of any information or suggestions in this book.

Archway Publishing books may be ordered through booksellers or by contacting:

Archway Publishing
1663 Liberty Drive
Bloomington, IN 47403
www.archwaypublishing.com
1 (888) 242-5904

Because of the dynamic nature of the Internet, any web addresses or links contained in this book may have changed since publication and may no longer be valid. The views expressed in this work are solely those of the author and do not necessarily reflect the views of the publisher, and the publisher hereby disclaims any responsibility for them.

Any people depicted in stock imagery provided by Getty Images are models, and such images are being used for illustrative purposes only.
Certain stock imagery © Getty Images.

ISBN: 978-1-4808-7572-2 (sc)
ISBN: 978-1-4808-7573-9 (hc)
ISBN: 978-1-4808-7571-5 (e)

Library of Congress Control Number: 2019906881

Print information available on the last page.

Archway Publishing rev. date: 6/6/2019

CONTENTS

ACKNOWLEDGMENTS

Thank you to all the people I've met in my travels of life over the years, some of whom I have kept in touch with, some of whom I have put into this book, and some of whom have changed the trajectory of my life. Without you, I would not be here now, writing these words.

My readers, thank you for believing enough and having the confidence to read this book. Without you, I would not be here now, writing these words.

Thank you to my health science expert, Amber Landsman, MSc. I have felt fortunate to be working with you. Without you, I would not be here now, writing these words.

And finally, to my daughter Dana and to Shari, Lisa, Jeff, Amy, Eddie, Bobby, and Charlie—thank you for your patience, support, and love. You are the ones I travel with now. Thank you for bringing into my heart the perfect orchestration of the symphony of my life. Without you, I would not be here now, writing these words.

Love you all.

FOREWORD

As the author of the book **Your Best Age is Now**, I know how important it is to reboot your life, especially during middle age. For anyone looking to achieve feeling their best at any age, they not only need to do the right correctional emotional work, they also need to take better care of themselves, particularly when it comes to their health.

When our hormones are out of balance it can cause disturbing disruptions. Hormones are powerful chemicals in our bodies that keep our bodies functioning normally. The word hormone is derived from the Greek word hormo which means to set in motion.

Whether you are dealing with PMS or Menopause, hormones can affect everything from your weight, self-esteem, sex drive to your food cravings. These hormone fluctuations can make women feel overwhelmed and like they are losing control of their lives.

Extensive research shows an association between decreased levels of estrogen and progesterone causing everything from depression, anxiety and mood swings especially as a woman becomes peri-menopausal. And these symptoms can increase and intensify even further during menopause.

Other symptoms include:

- foggy mind
- hot flashes
- memory lapses, and
- headaches.

Experts advise women to pay close attention to maintaining a healthy weight during this time, which means learning how to pay close attention to both your eating habits and exercise. While we may not be able to change our genetics, we can change our lifestyle. And this lifestyle change can have a favorable impact on our hormones. Even after menopause, there can be some level of reproductive hormones in the body which can cause symptoms of depression, anxiety or mild mood swings, years beyond a woman's last period.

The great news is there are a lot of things women can do to take back control of their emotional health and life. There are answers for every woman at every stage. Women no longer have to feel victimized by haywire hormones. And for many the answers lie in the diet, natural herbs and supplements they use.

For a growing number of ladies, B3H+ is the next, most logical step for them to take in order to help them care for themselves, their health and their bodies.

B3H+ is a science-based medically supervised breakthrough weight loss program which has helped many midlife women achieve their weight loss goals while also helping them live their best life. The testimonials are quite impressive! Women who have embraced the program, have rediscovered their sexy, healthy selves and are approaching life with a Joie De Vivre, living every moment like, **Your Best Age is Now.**

-Dr. Robi Ludwig (psychotherapist, author & TV commentator)

PREFACE

With this book, I hope to convey to all women struggling with weight loss that it doesn't have to be a struggle, and you certainly don't have to go through it alone. Here at the Balance 3H Plus centers we pride ourselves in finding the underlying causes of your weight gain and weight loss resistance. We then devise integrative and natural solutions to correct those issues so you have true, sustainable weight loss. Above all, we make sure you are not alone on your journey. While we encourage clients to take the reins of their own health and well-being, we are always here for support.

Even though weight loss is our specialty, I want women to understand that weight loss success is about much more than before-and-after pictures, achieving that "bikini body", or seeing the number on the scale go down.

It's about the small victories and the quiet triumphs, such as being able to breath easier, sleep deeper, having the energy to play with your children or grandchildren, travel the world, or dancing the night away. It's about having the confidence to wear that fitted dress again or shine brightly in conversations with friends, family members or new acquaintances. Weight loss is also about improving your overall health and well-being. As you already know, health is the most valuable type of wealth. When you have your health, the quality of your life improves exponentially—and this is my ultimate wish for you!

Mitchell R. Suss
CEO Balance 3H Plus
www.Balance3HPlus.com

ABOUT BALANCE 3H PLUS

Balance 3H Plus (B3H+) was created by physicians with the help of other health experts as a new medically supervised, weight-loss program for women.

B3H+ is a science-based program specifically for women who are in perimenopause and menopause, ages forty to sixty-five.

If you ever experienced hormonal changes that resulted in symptoms such as weight gain, skin issues, digestive problems, sleep disorders, mood swings, fatigue, or thyroid issues, then your hormones are probably not balanced.

B3H+ is an all-natural, metabolism-and-hormone-focused program that helps women of all shapes and sizes naturally balance their hormones to stimulate fat loss and recapture their youth.

Excess fat (especially around the waist) is what causes many hormonal imbalances, and the B3H+ program can repair those imbalances.

B3H+ is a program built upon the unique physiology of the female body. The program helps women adopt a healthier way of eating that enhances their metabolism, decreases inflammation in the body, and works to boost energy levels.

Women should find it easy to use and sustainable, meaning not only will they see results, but they will be able to keep the weight off for good. All without having to eat less and exercise more.

INTRODUCTION

Getting serious about your health is a wonderful and immensely rewarding gift to yourself. Remaining fit in the season of middle age becomes more difficult. Perhaps you're frustrated and need some encouragement. Or maybe you want guidance from someone you can trust, who won't steer you wrong. You've tried every fad diet and exercise trend, but your body is not responding. Things that used to work to keep you fit and lean just don't anymore. The harder you try, the more it seems to fail you. Guess what? It's not your fault!

The truth is, your weight, eating habits, and health are not a result of laziness, gluttony, lack of willpower, or consistency at the gym. You have become trapped inside a body that is not functioning well and needs special attention and repair. There is no combination of dieting, willpower, physical activity, psychotherapy, and pep talks that can give your body the help it needs. You need an entirely new, revolutionary approach to reveal what is going on inside your body, and to deal with the unique changes women encounter in midlife. You need a holistic approach, one that includes a safe, effective, nature-based biochemical overhaul.

This is not going to be like any other book you have ever read about diet, aging, and health. It will not tell you how many calories to eat or what percentages of macronutrients you need. It won't tell you that you don't have enough discipline, willpower, or are too lazy to stick with a diet plan. Neither will it tell you that your slow metabolism, mood swings, food cravings, or deteriorating health are just circumstances you should accept as part of growing older.

The shift into midlife allows you great opportunity to go from proving your legitimacy to the world to artfully manifesting and living your legacy. You see, you can still feel as lively, smart, strong, sexy, and even more relevant in your forties, fifties, and sixties—and beyond—as you were in your twenties and early thirties. I already know what you're thinking: *Are you kidding me? The media glorifies only the young, and as gravity attacks my body, how am I supposed to feel that I can compete with millennial "it girls"?* Who said you have to? The only thing that you *must* do is take care of your health, and *never give up!*

It has become my life's mission to help people look and feel biologically younger and to live more vibrantly. I understand what you're going through. I've spent much of my life struggling with my own weight and have had to fight for good health. I have great compassion for women experiencing the same thing.

When I was a young boy, my mother was diagnosed with a terminal form of cancer. As her primary caretaker, I watched her teeter back and forth between moments of pain, frustration, and sadness, and moments of optimism and spiritual strength. I was there with her and all of her emotional highs and lows until she passed.

This time with my mother taught me how delicate and fleeting life can be. It taught me how to become a man with an open, compassionate heart and to explore deep, authentic connections with other women whom I would come to love and care for. I have since walked through the emotional highs and lows this season of life brings with my ex-wife and other close friends, and I have made it my life's purpose to do something to help all of us.

I have come to understand that all women desire emotional understanding and open communication in relationships, but often struggle to find it. It's hard to talk about hormonal changes, especially when you don't really understand what's happening. Many women over forty develop "out of nowhere" muffin tops, general weight gain, chronic pains, wild mood swings, and feelings of fatigue, anxiety, depression, and hopelessness at the thought of dieting forever just to stay lean. I did not want this frustration and downward cycle of poor health to cloud over one more woman. I began searching to find the keys to unlock the secrets of harmonious healthy aging and the hidden causes of midlife weight gain, weight loss resistance, and hormonal havoc. It would take me along with Dr. Siobhan Kealy a well-informed, patient, supportive women's health doctor years of research to decode the most challenging obstacles to midlife weight loss, and to achieving a sustainable, internal balance and external transformation.

In 2015, Dr. Kealy and I decided to open the medical weight-loss center, Balance 3H Plus (hereinafter referred to as B3H+, Balance 3H Plus, or the Program). We assembled a team of physicians, functional nutritionists, and women's health experts who could focus on getting clients to take back their health. Our goal was to offer entirely new solutions that would help them to feel better in and about their bodies, end middle-age weight gain, and live younger longer.

One thing I came across in our research was the life expectancy statistics for both men and women. I saw that women were easily outliving men by five or more years, and for a variety of theoretical reasons. Although the scientific explanations are not yet definitive, there is a strong show of support for both the genetic and hormonal differences helping women live longer. However, regardless of where women's biological survival advantage is coming from, my findings reinforced a long-held belief of mine that women are made for longevity. Women possess a robust variety of inherent traits like empathy, resiliency, ferocity, compassion, curiosity, attention to detail, and undying passion. These traits empower them to thrive for long periods of time in demanding careers, at home, and in close relationships, and just maybe in living well and living longer.

I asked myself, *How can I help women who are already using their Superwoman-like inherent traits to quickly and safely achieve their optimal health and body weight and find grace and peace in aging?* Women just like *you* inspired my original idea of the medical weight-loss program, Balance 3H Plus. This program is a holistic, total wellness plan. It has helped thousands of women who have felt hopeless, fat, ashamed, scared, and unwanted to enjoy health and longevity. The Program is specifically designed to provide you with the steps to overcome midlife hormonal havoc that can lead directly to food cravings, overeating, and unnecessary weight gain. We intend to free you permanently from the intense cravings, the diet mentality, and food obsessions. Soon you'll instinctively be eating in ways that are aligned with your female genetics and metabolic hormones. You'll also be integrating physical and restorative practices that help you reboot and refresh. We will help you rebalance your body chemistry *naturally* so you can attain your optimal weight and health—for good.

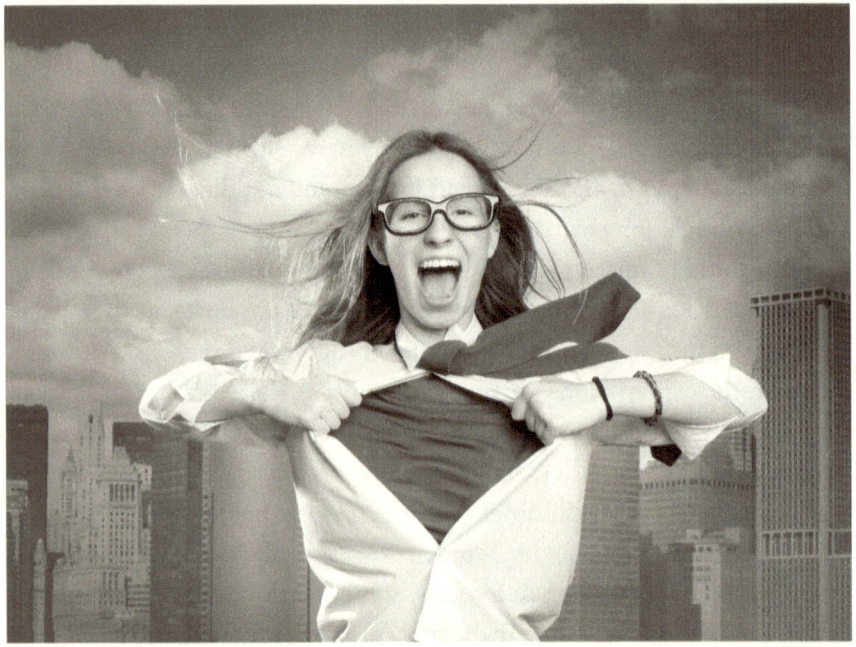

Our Balance 3H Plus experts look at every client as a friend as they confer support, empathy, confidentiality, and love. Our caring approach gives rise to mutual respect, trust, and understanding, which are desperately needed in the world today. We seem to have lost sight of this power of personal connection—a connection that can motivate, empower, and give people with all types of adversities the ability to cope, build on their resiliency, and thrive. We connect with each client differently in order to provide a uniquely formulated program of support, medically through metabolic blood panels and natural therapies as well as nutritionally, emotionally, and physically. Our clients end up feeling younger, healthier, more energetic, and they end up looking sexier and leaner. Best of all, they come away from our program armed with the education and body awareness they need so they can respond to and resolve every situation without harming their delicately balanced metabolism.

Women who come to Balance 3H Plus centers are encouraged to share their deeply personal health stories and weight struggles with us and with one another. This creates an atmosphere of mutual support, understanding, and compassion, which increases their desire to pursue their optimal health and well-being. The key to your success is that we believe we have uncovered a missing ingredient in the soup of perpetual health. It's not enough to provide valid and reliable health information with solutions for real results. We need to offer women continuous support so they can naturally connect with other women and feel safe when communicating fears, insecurities, frustrations, and lessons in order to sustain the changes she makes and wants in life.

References Introduction:

1. Eskes, T., Haanen C., "Why do women live longer than men?" *European Journal of Obstetrics & Gynecology and Reproductive Biology.* Volume 133, Issue 2, (2007) 126–133.
2. Waldron I., "Sex Differences in Human Mortality: The role of genetic factors," *Social Science & Medicine,* Volume 17, Issue 6 (1983), 321–333.

CHAPTER 1
IT'S NOT YOUR FAULT

My friend, Vicky, is fifty-one and has been through it all—marriage, parenthood, caring for ailing parents, unemployment, and divorce—but she has always appeared calm, focused, and self-confident while navigating life's unexpected challenges. She has exhibited resiliency, strength, and determination as well as deep love and devotion for family members, friends, and a demanding career. Vicky seemed to be acutely aware of her feelings and able to transform and dissolve tension quickly, enabling her to return to a relaxed state of mind.

One Sunday afternoon three years ago, we met for lunch. After checking in briefly, we settled into an open but unusually serious and unsettling conversation. She started complaining to me about everything—her body shape, skin imperfections, joint problems, lack of motivation to exercise, and even the people in her close circle. At that moment, she was in attack mode toward herself and others. I lacked the courage to temper her frustration and anger. Her criticisms seemed completely unwarranted, she lacked focus, her confidence seemed shaken, and her thinking seemed irrational and self-deprecating. *What is causing her so much emotional distress?* I thought to myself. *She's obviously suffering from something that's making her feel unstable and awful about herself and life.* As I continued to listen to one negative statement after another, I realized my close friend's heart, body, and mind were being hijacked without her even realizing it. Then, within a space of a few minutes, she went from angry and frustrated

1

to embarrassed. She sobbed hysterically as she talked about her core needs and feelings of being ignored and devalued by others. She felt invisible as a middle-aged women. She could no longer suffer her mood swings in silence; it had become too painful. Vicky was also struggling to get enough sleep due to severe night sweats, and this was, without a doubt, affecting her mood. She was experiencing brain fog, fatigue, bouts of anxiety, and steady weight gain. It seemed as though every aspect of her familiar, younger years of well-being were outside her reach. She left me that day seeming hopeless, frustrated, embarrassed, and unlovable. What Vicky was going through was menopause, and what she didn't know is that it was not her fault—it was her hormones.

Ultimately, Vicky's challenges with menopausal symptoms inspired me to research and learn extensively about hormone imbalances in middle-aged women. I wanted to be able to help her and others like her rebalance their hormones and, by extension, their metabolism and quality of life.

Midlife Hormonal Imbalances: The Hidden Culprit

Today women spend decades building their professional legitimacy while balancing relationships, motherhood, care-giving to ailing parents, and a full social calendar. They are expected to manage all of that as if they were endowed with superhuman powers and endless youth. However, all women, to differing degrees, experience the unpleasant symptoms that come with aging. The multitasking they once performed with confidence and ease becomes nearly impossible as the effects of perimenopause—and eventually, menopause—set in.

The discomforts and uncertainties of modern hormonal imbalances, which so many middle-aged women suffer from, are overwhelming their spirits and negatively affecting their sleep, energy, focus, motivation, and relationships. In addition, and often most devastatingly, their metabolism slows, excess weight appears overnight, sugar cravings become uncontrollable, and a whole host of adverse symptoms and other health conditions can develop.

The dreaded discomforts of this change of life show up in some not-so-obvious areas too. Many women over the age of fifty report that, as they age, they feel as if the women they've always felt to be seems to vanish. They feel as if they are being replaced by old, easily-forgettable women, no longer seen as desirable or attractive. It's as if they have been transported back in time to the "nerdiest," most awkward, and horrifyingly embarrassing moments in high school. In reality, teen years, with their goofy growth spurts, pimples, and greasy skin, and middle age, with its weight gain, wrinkles, and saggy skin, are both marked by waves of hormones, mood swings, irrational reactions to social situations, and hyper-awareness of appearance.

So how, then, can women like Vicky rebalance their hormones and restore their good health during perimenopause and menopause? What natural things can they do with exercise, targeted supplements, bioidentical hormones, and nutrition? My goal with this book is to provide you with answers to these common questions, answers that address the real issues and causes of unbalanced hormones and aim to stop the vicious cycle of menopausal symptoms.

My Story, My Intentions, My Philosophy

The first things people notice about me are my large frame and my larger-than-life character. I have always been a person who seems to gain weight by just looking at fattening foods—or any food for that matter. Fluctuations in my weight were as frequent as the sunrise. But they were not the normal weight fluctuations that most people see on the scale from meal to meal and day to day, which, as frustrating as they are, are normal and usually temporary and happen to everyone. These weight fluctuations are typically caused by factors such as consumption of a big meal, high salt intake, water retention, or "consti-poop-tion." That's why most nutritionists discourage weighing ourselves daily. Unfortunately, my weight fluctuations were only going in one direction—up. Sadly, my weight continued to creep in this singular direction from childhood into adulthood. I struggled to find a balanced weight.

I was quite unaware of the long-term health consequences of my poor food choices. They were changing more than just what my body looked like on the outside. The large portions and sugary and fatty foods were giving me a short-term reward but destroying my health and interrupting my hormones, particularly my testosterone level. I was caught in a cycle of poor eating that created a cascade of chemical, physical, and even emotional stress. I lived like this for years and felt lousy, unmotivated, and uncommitted to change.

I have a witty sense of humor (or so I'm told), so I naturally put a comedic spin on my weight situation. I would say things like, "Hey, the more I weigh, the harder I am to kidnap!" My humor and sarcasm made my friends laugh, but I knew this self-deprecating, unhealthy talk reflected a tight lid on my true feelings and fears about changing. There was nothing funny about the years that I endured trying to uncover the information and help I desperately needed.

My hormones and brain chemistry were totally *wacked!* I knew I had a long road of body restoration and reprogramming ahead of me. Although I had no idea where to start, what kind of questions to ask, or what sort of experts to consult, I knew it was time to begin my healing journey. I wanted to get out of the toxic food and diet mentality and "Get Back into Living Again," as music legend Curtis Mayfield's classic hit from *New World Order* declares. I was ready to rebalance my mind and body chemistry and end the food cravings, weight gain, and mood swings—naturally. I was finally on my way to reclaiming my health in order to lose the weight for good.

Shortly after I made this decision, I found my endocrinologist, who ordered multiple hormone tests. The tests showed my testosterone levels were in the tank. Testosterone is an important muscle-building and fat-loss-enhancing hormone. My endocrinologist prescribed a personalized dose of natural testosterone and suggested several supportive supplements, an exercise program, and other natural ways for me to recover. Within weeks, my hormone levels balanced and I started to lose the fat. Several short months later, I had lost thirty pounds of *fat mass*, not just weight on the scale.

It's been ten years since I started using hormone replacement therapy and bioidentical supplements, eating a whole-food diet, exercising, and using other natural remedies to maintain a healthy weight. The greatest thing is, I really don't miss any of those foods I used to eat. I no longer have insatiable cravings, am starving between meals, or the desire for the same "old" foods. I have much more energy. I feel better than ever about my weight, and I am now able to recognize non-hunger-related eating habits swiftly. Now I eat to live—to live my authentic purpose.

A Dream Solution—The Balance 3H Plus Program

One night, I had surreal dream in which everyone was eating frosted cakes, gourmet pies, and tasty pastries, but they all looked lean, fit, and healthy. This dream made me think that people probably would like to have their cake and lose fat too, as I always did. But this, I knew from personal experience, was no formula for real health. The crazy dream fed my inspiration to help others and motivated me to get the message out about how hormonal imbalances play a key role in middle-aged weight gain and weight-loss resistance.

The story of my personal experiences, struggles, and then success with my weight and hormones was the exact message that I wanted to get out to the world. I wanted to open everyone's eyes to the power of balancing hormones in order to change their bodies and overall wellness. This was a new, sustainable method to restore total health and boost aging, sluggish metabolism to lose unwanted fat forever.

This approach to reprogramming our body chemistries had to be based in valid scientific research with proven clinical results. It had to combine the latest research in nutritional biochemistry, endocrinology, neurochemistry, psychology, physiology, exercise science, and alternative health sciences. And most importantly, it had to consider a person's unique genetics, lifestyle, personal preferences, health history, habits, and metabolic needs. I needed to develop a program that could forever change the body's fat-burning physiology.

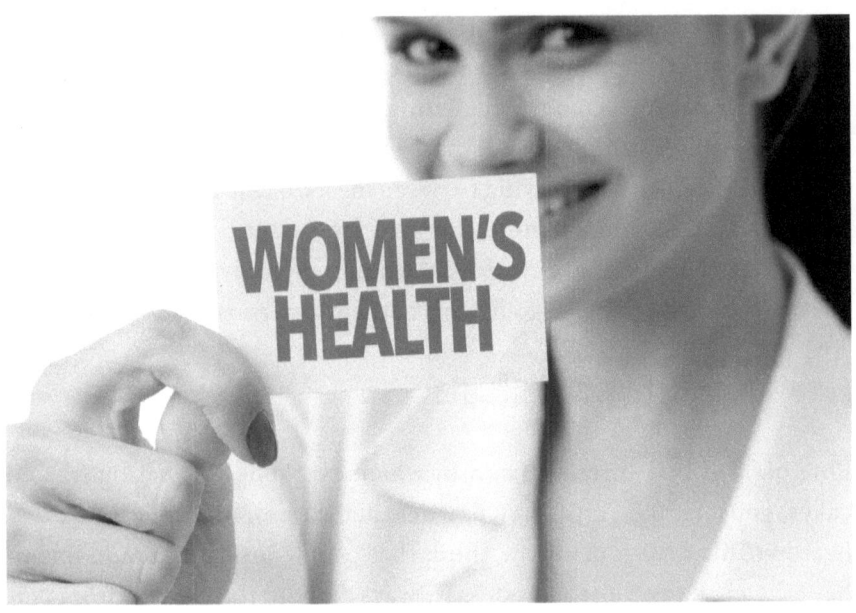

Late in 2015, I put my smaller frame and still larger-than-life character to good use as an ambassador and advocate of our revolutionary medical weight-loss program, Balance 3H Plus. I did this so people just like me—and you—never have to diet again. The genesis of this program comes directly from my personal experiences. My lifelong challenge has also inspired and motivated me to write this book, so people know that being fat is not their fault; neither is it their fate. Aging and time should make us wiser, not necessarily wider. By combining the information in this book with our program, you will learn habits that will quickly result in getting back the figure and metabolism of your youth.

I truly believe we deserve the opportunity to learn extensively, if we choose, about what's under the hood of our one and only vehicle. At B3H+ centers, we offer our clients a workable, customized, holistic template for how their bodies work best and how they respond to different internal and external stimuli such as foods, stress, sleep, and so forth. So much of what many of us have learned about how our bodies work isn't wholly accurate. Many of us are having to retrain our minds and bodies. Thus, an important feature and focus of the Balance 3H Plus Program is creating a road map of alternative treatments, simple techniques, and tools that you can learn and easily apply to get your desired results.

Healing and Treating *You*, Not Just Symptoms

Early on in life, most people are taught to go to their medicine cabinets and reach for pill bottles in order to control symptoms or even resolve health issues. A doctor's word is often considered sacrosanct, immune to questioning. Evaluating and treating the causes of symptoms, the individual, and the ability to *prevent* conditions are often subordinated to the immediacy of alleviating symptoms by way of prescription drugs such as synthetic hormones, stimulants, benzodiazepines (for anxiety), or antidepressants. The harmful effects of long-term use, misuse, or abuse of such medications is shocking. Long-term use often leads to more serious disorders, more diseases, and sometimes more deaths than those resulting from firearms and motor vehicle accidents.

We genuinely want to help unlock what your body needs and guide you along your own path toward healthy living. We're committed to helping you ultimately achieve the balance you deserve and desire, both hormonally and in life during this transformation. The B3H+ Program keeps a close watch on current research discoveries in women's health so that we can respond by offering you the most effective, natural, lasting solutions to hormonal imbalances. In doing so, we recognize that our weight-loss program and wellness services work best when our clients remain open to shifting away from the diet mindset and to learning our new sustainable approach to weight management. You, as the client, must be willing to actively investigate for yourself so you better understand the application and solutions that work for your unique metabolism, genetics, psychology, and personal preferences. We've created the B3H+ Program, but it won't work without your commitment to making the lifestyle changes required to keep you healthy and youthful.

It's up to you to say, "*Yes!* I want my life to be as abundantly healthy, vibrant, and enjoyable as possible for many years to come!" The Program will be so much more effective if we can work together as a team in learning key strategies, teaching you how to apply them, and answering your questions as you *grow and go*. Our program offers you a time-and money-saving investment that pays dividends in good health, a sexier and more fit body, sustained energy, and hormonal harmony.

How the B3H+ Program Worked for Me

Name: Amy

Age: 55

Starting weight: 301 pounds

Total weight lost: 71 pounds

Current weight: 230 pounds

Beyond exhausted is how I felt after ten years as the full-time caregiver to my elderly parents. I felt totally disconnected from the outside world, isolated, and burned out. I suffered from night sweats, disturbed sleep, brain fog, and constant hunger. The B3H+ medical team and nutrition experts were compassionate and kind, and started a program for me immediately. They discovered I was deficient in several vitamins and minerals which impaired my metabolism and made it almost impossible for me to burn fat. Six months later, I feel energized, alive, reconnected with people, am seventy-one pounds lighter, and am living a life I love—and life is loving me back.

CHAPTER 2
BETTER TOGETHER

On my quest to find the best weight-loss specialists in the country and assemble a team of women's health experts, I discovered a smart, vibrant physician named Dr. Siobhan Kealy. Educated in endocrine health and nutrition, Dr. Kealy had worked in this area for decades, offering women nutrition coaching and customized fitness programs to help them lose weight and reclaim their health and vitality. After working with hundreds of patients each year, Dr. Kealy realized it was nearly impossible for perimenopausal and menopausal women to lose weight and feel great just through diet and exercise. A healthy diet and adequate amounts of exercise alone were not addressing the underlying cause of unwanted weight gain—hormonal imbalances.

So Dr. Kealy and my team of medical weight-loss experts partnered with each other and began our crusade for answers to better understand how women's hormones impact their weight and health during perimenopause and menopause. We discovered that midlife hormonal imbalances not only contribute to a women's inability to lose weight, but also affect their mood, sleep, skin, joints, energy, appetite, and rate of aging.

Our newly formed partnership led to the creation of the B3H+ Program, which addresses many of the barriers to losing weight after age forty. The B3H+ Program was born out of a need to fill the gaps between the one-size-fits-all diet industry, the hormone replacement industry, and the medical community.

Together, we follow our passion of giving women hope, knowledge, life-changing scientifically supported solutions, and a new direction to "heal thyself" so they can get their weight, energy, and optimism where they have always wanted them to be!

• • •

Meet Dr. Siobhan Kealy!

All across America, I am known as a women's health expert, speaker, and radio and TV personality. But first and foremost, I am a woman. And like you, I know what it feels like to be fighting fatigue and midlife weight gain, mood swings, belly bloat, and a lower libido.

For over twenty years, I have been helping women change and revolutionize their health, body weight, and lives. When women come to me, they are often overweight, fatigued, stressed, depressed, and in pain. The diet industry has deceived them and failed them again and again. And their yo-yo, crash dieting past, in addition to stress and less activity, has only worsened their chronic inflammation, hormonal imbalances, aches, pains, and sluggish metabolism.

Are you entering your forties? Are you eating less and exercising more? How many diets have you tried—five, ten, twenty? Countless diets promise you the body you have always wanted. You have strictly followed these diet plans only to end up weighing more than you did when you started. And, ultimately, you feel like a failure and a fool for buying into another diet scam.

If this sounds like you, then maybe you are ready to take my challenge. I challenge you to stop dieting and start balancing! Yes, you heard me correct, *stop* dieting!

In this science-based, medical weight-loss program, I offer you a natural, safe solution to counteract the dreadful symptoms of menopause.

So what's the secret to staying slim, sane, and sexy after forty?

Balancing hormones! This three-phase program includes hormonal testing and rebalancing, a gentle detoxification, a sensible eating plan (not another diet), and nutraceutical supplements for additional nutrients and metabolic support. Also included are lifestyle strategies and an age-appropriate exercise program. (Yes, you should exercise differently after forty.)

The simple fact is that many middle-aged women find themselves in a place where they need an extra metabolic boost in order to start losing weight. In this program, we help block further fat storage, increase your metabolism, and improve your fat-burning potential. Although, what really sets us apart from everyone else is that we work with you to rebalance hormones, reset your adrenal glands, and decrease systemic inflammation. There is also research to suggest that balancing women's hormones helps reduce the risk of heart disease and prevents certain hormone-sensitive cancers.

To determine a woman's hormone levels, I created the industry's most comprehensive blood test panel for women, appropriately named Health 365. It is the first of its kind to use mathematical analysis of DNA and hormones. With a Health 365 report, I can analyze the genetic markers and blood values that make up your body chemistry, and I can isolate imbalances and their underlying cause. Then we deliver you a customized report and reveal the next steps for living the healthy and vibrant life you desire.

Would you like to experience these kinds of health changes in your life?

If you answer yes, then I am here to tell you that you are in the right place. You do not have to "grin and

bear it" and "power through" perimenopause and menopause like most women do. It is not your fault; it is your
hormones!

It is possible to reverse and prevent the effects of aging, including weight gain and disease. You can look and
feel amazing at age forty—and beyond.

Sound good? Then let's begin!

I'd like to share a few stories—real stories from real
women:

My patient, **Melanie**, forty-five, initially came to
me when she began to notice a slow but steady weight
gain. We talked, tested her hormones and thyroid, but
she wasn't committed to changing her lifestyle and diet.
A year later, she had gained an additional seven pounds.
Over the course of this time period, she had not changed
her diet or her exercise routine. Melanie certainly wasn't
obese, and most of her friends family members did not
even notice the weight change, but she certainly did. Her
shirts were snugger around the middle, and her pants were
tighter around her bum. This weight gain with no valid
explanation really bothered her, and she became terrified
of packing on more pounds. Therefore, Melanie returned
to my clinic ready to commit to transforming her life.

First, I tested for imbalanced hormones. I was able to
analyze her personal genetic markers and isolate imbalances and their underlying causes. Her tests also indicated
blood sugar abnormalities (a high A1C marker), which
was a key factor in her weight gain. With all this new information, we uncovered the primary causes of her weight
problem. Together, we customized a hormone balancing
program that was tailored to her needs, age, and body
chemistry. After two months on the Program she lost the
seven pounds she had gained, plus a few more. Today she
feels she has a new lease on life. As a doctor in practice for

over twenty years, I have learned that the world is full of frustrated menopausal women just like Melanie.

Now meet **Ann**, age forty-nine. She went from feeling frustrated to feeling fabulous. She was a brilliant CEO of a high-profile financial company. Ann's dietary and lifestyle habits in her twenties and early thirties caused several hormonal imbalances and health problems. She had chronic sugar and food cravings, endometriosis, hypothyroidism, and mild depression. Ann was constantly struggling to change things on her own with a "healthy" but restrictive diet and harder, longer exercise sessions. Of course, none of this was helping Ann, and most of it was only causing further imbalances and health issues. Fortunately, I was able to restore her body to health and reset her hormones. What's more, she lost a tremendous amount of weight—a total of twenty-five pounds over three short months. Ann's story is truly inspirational. Now she shares her B3H+ Program experience and how she regained her health and her life!

Meet **Ellen,** fifty-two, the mother of three teenage daughters. She was a complete wreck at her first visit. At fifty-two, she was nearing menopause and had irregular periods. She also suffered from chronic depression, for which she had been prescribed several antidepressants over the last ten years. Ellen had attempted unsuccessfully to lose weight numerous times. She had tried many of the popular diet programs including Jenny Craig, Weight Watchers, and the Atkins diet.

Ellen advised me that she was too lethargic to exercise. She also experienced persistent sadness, cried frequently, and continually gained weight and retained water (a symptom associated with progesterone deficiency). She had out-of-control cravings for sugar and could not control her appetite.

Ellen's problems were due to her hormones being out of balance. Our comprehensive blood test revealed Ellen was low in estrogen, progesterone, and dehydroepiandrosterone (DHEA). Her stress hormone cortisol was high, and hunger hormones leptin and ghrelin were out of whack.

Many of you may be familiar with Ellen's situation. Most women going through perimenopause or menopause experience a host of symptoms: hot flashes, fatigue, night sweats, mood swings, and weight gain.

I started Ellen on a customized version of the B3H+ Program. After two months, she lost nineteen pounds and reported that her moods had stabilized; in fact, her primary doctor began tapering off her antidepressants. Her energy has improved dramatically. She now exercises three times a week and continues to lose weight. As you can see by Ellen's transformation, weight problems caused by imbalanced hormones can be improved significantly on the B3H+ Program.

Finally, I have experience with my own middle age health and hormones challenges and dissatisfactions. I gained a belly bulge after hitting forty and found myself feeling daily aches and pains in my joints. I was also not recovering as quickly from my workouts as I did when I was in my twenties and thirties. Fortunately, this became even a greater motivator for me to delve deeper into the research surrounding the biological effects and changes women go through after forty.

I hope these examples show you that no matter what your history, life circumstances, or amount of weight you need to lose, you can successfully lose the fat—forever!

Dr. Siobhan Kealy
Creator and Medical Director, B3H+

CHAPTER 3
UNDERSTANDING HORMONES

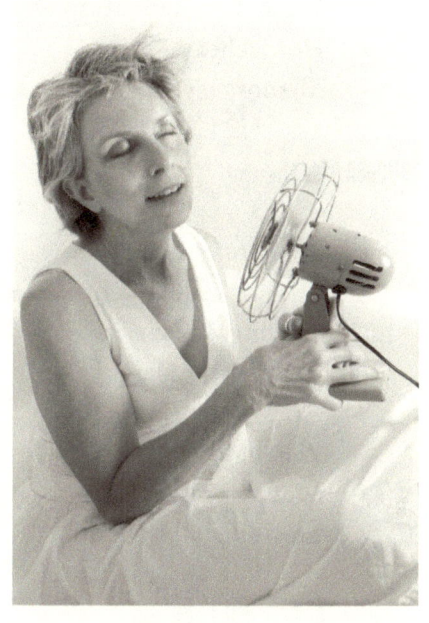

As I mentioned, hormone imbalances affect virtually every life-giving function, as well as longevity. When hormones are imbalanced, a total body disruption occurs. Below is a quick summary of some of the most common hormones tested along with the major symptoms that arise when they are out of balance. By testing the levels of these hormones, we gain crucial information regarding deficiencies, excesses, and daily patterns. The results enable us to specifically tailor a treatment approach for each individual.

The major sex hormones to assess are: estrogen, progesterone, and testosterone. The main adrenal hormones are DHEA (a precursor to estrogen and testosterone) and cortisol. Additionally, thyroid hormone is a critical metabolic manager.

Hormone imbalances affect estrogen, progesterone, testosterone,

DHEA, cortisol, and thyroid hormones. These imbalances can manifest themselves in one or more ways:

Estrogen deficiency

- Hot flashes
- Depression
- Sleep disturbances
- Dry skin
- Foggy thinking
- Heart palpitations
- Night sweats
- Vaginal dryness/atrophy
- Headaches
- Memory lapses

Estrogen excess

- Water retention
- Breast swelling/tenderness
- Cravings for sweets
- Heavy, irregular menses
- Fatigue
- Weight gain
- Mood swings
- Low-thyroid symptoms

Progesterone deficiency

- Swollen breasts
- Headaches
- Anxiety
- Irregular menstrual cycle
- Cramping

- Weight gain
- Low libido
- Mood swings
- Depression
- PMS
- Bone Loss
- Water retention

Progesterone excess

- Somnolence (sleepiness, drowsiness)
- Mild depression
- Candida (yeast overgrowth)
- Bloating
- Breast swelling
- Exacerbation of estrogen deficiency
- Constipation, loose stools, or a combination of both

Testosterone deficiency

- Abdominal fat
- Difficulty losing fat
- Fatigue
- Reduced muscle mass
- Memory problems
- Low libido
- Bone loss
- Facial hair
- Depression, mood swings, anxiety
- Thinning skin
- Vaginal dryness
- General aches and pains
- Insomnia

Testosterone excess

- Poly cystic ovarian syndrome (PCOS)
- Loss of scalp hair
- Increased body and facial hair
- Oily skin
- Irregular menstrual cycle

DHEA deficiency

- Lower estrogen production
- Changes in immune system function (accelerates aging and disease risk, such as cancer)

High DHEA excess

- Higher testosterone levels
- Higher insulin levels
- Higher risk for polycystic ovary syndrome (PCOS)

Cortisol deficiency (not very common)

- Fatigue
- Low libido
- Immunocompromised
- Cravings for salty foods
- Chemical sensitivities
- Symptoms of low progesterone
- Allergies
- Irritability
- Symptoms of hypothyroidism

Cortisol excess (too common)

- Abdominal fat
- Cravings for starch and sweets
- Increased hunger
- Erratic energy levels
- Reduced muscle mass
- Bone loss
- Sleep disturbances
- Low libido
- Anxiety
- Depression
- Scalp hair loss

Thyroid Hormone deficiency (too common)

- Slow metabolism
- Fatigue (especially evening)
- Cold sensitivity
- Low libido
- Dry skin
- General aches and pains
- Depression
- Scalp hair loss
- Brittle nails
- Low pulse rate and blood pressure
- Memory lapses
- Heart palpitations
- Low stamina
- Low body temperature
- Headaches
- Anxiety
- Swollen, puffy eyes
- Decreased swelling

- Poor concentration
- High cholesterol
- Infertility

Thyroid Hormone Excess (much less common)

- Nervousness or anxiety
- Skin dryness
- Excessive sweating
- Weight loss
- Sleep problems
- Heart rate changes
- Increased bowel movements
- Hand tremors
- Weakness

If you have experienced any of these symptoms, don't despair. We have nutritional, medical, and fitness experts on our staff who have been educated in conventional medicine, as well as the functional medical practices of endocrinology, nutritional biochemistry, stress management, and exercise science. Their combined educational and research experiences have obtained positive results for thousands of clients, eliminating the causes of their symptoms and changing their metabolisms and hormones *naturally.*

A natural method is the use of bioidentical hormones, which are identical to the hormones that women make in their bodies—also called "natural hormones."

The physical and emotional changes experienced by women during perimenopause and menopause are often misdiagnosed and, in some instances, even considered psychological in nature. There is so much misinformation about perimenopause and menopause, most of which comes from less-informed practitioners, the media, drug companies, and "snake oil salesmen" who want to sell you something and play on your worst fears.

We often tell our clients, "It's not your momma's menopause!" You do not have to go through the difficult experiences your mother had transitioning into menopause or during menopause. Today, there is an array of natural remedies and treatment options available to help you cope and, better yet, thrive. They are much safer and often more effective at diminishing discomfort and distressing symptoms quickly. These methods include quality vitamins, supplements (nutraceuticals, which are supplements derived from food sources which provide health and medicinal benefits to the body), botanicals, bioidentical hormones, and other natural forms of hormone therapy and non-hormonal medications.

There is no reason for you to have to struggle and suffer. Remember: *It's not your fault; it's your hormones.* We pride ourselves in helping every woman enhance the quality of her health and life. Can we give women a dyed-in-the-wool solution to menopausal distress? No, but I would be so bold as to say that we have developed a highly effective option for most. For those who experience both the insidious and obvious symptoms during this midlife transition, our treatment programs offer real solutions and real results for every women. We believe that, with our unremitting attitudes, hard work, and dedication to our deepest purpose (which is improving *your* health and vitality), we will continue to bring women the latest solutions for lasting change.

On this ever-changing journey toward optimal wellness, we must take a closer look at the number-one preoccupation and cause of distress of women in midlife: challenges with weight maintenance and permanent fat loss.

Why It's Not Your Fault; It's Your Hormones

Unfortunately, many of us do not realize the impact that hormones have on our well-being and overall health. Hormones, which are your body's metabolic messengers, can be thought of as signaling molecules (in other words, chemical messengers) released by your cells, which influence every bodily function. For instance, a single imbalance of one or more hormones, can wreak havoc on things such as your thyroid or adrenal gland function, mood-enhancing brain chemicals, blood sugar levels, metabolism (your ability to use fat for fuel), or immune system. Particularly during middle age, women experience these dramatic hormonal changes causing intolerable perimenopausal and menopausal symptoms. We, however, want you to remember that there are safe, natural ways to treat these hormonal issues at any age, and *you don't have to suffer.*

Finding an optimal diet consisting of real, whole foods along with supplements and a lifestyle program to match your particular hormonal imbalances and relieve your adverse symptoms will make a world of difference in your menopausal experience.

Health 365

At Balance 3H Plus we offer our clients the industry's most comprehensive blood test panel for women, Health 365. It is the first of its kind to use mathematical analysis of DNA and hormones. With Health 365, Dr. Siobhan Kealy can analyze the genetic markers and blood values that make up your body chemistry, and isolate imbalances and their underlying cause.

Body chemistry is defined by a patient's unique genetically determined level of hormones, pre-hormones, vitamins, enzymes, proteins, and electrolytes. The variables in this complex ecosystem are all highly interdependent; even a small change in one can have dramatic effects on your ability to lose weight and sustain healthy habits. Our panel of tests is tailored specifically for women in their menopausal stages. Health 365 allows us to correctly identify and reset the hormones that are preventing you from looking, performing, and feeling your absolute best.

What does the Health 365 laboratory test analyze?

- Measures and analyzes broad panel-based biomolecules and DNA genetic markers
- Analyzes twenty blood base biomolecules, including cortisol (stress hormone), leptin (appetite suppressor hormone), ghrelin (hunger hormone), IGF-1,

DHEA-sulfate, follicle-stimulating hormone, testosterone, and estrodiol
- Analyzes fat soluble vitamins (A, D, E, and K), water soluble vitamins (B6, B9, B12, and C), minerals (calcium, magnesium, and potassium), hemoglobin A1C, heratocrit, and sex-hormone-binding hormone globulin
- Tests for key genetic mutations that impair how the body metabolizes certain hormones and vitamins that affect your ability to lose weight. A sample of these mutations include Factor V and the MTHFR gene
- Identifying these genetic mutations is imperative. Mutations can cause serious health risks and weight gain

There are approximately fifty hormones in the female body, but three are particularly crucial to perimenopausal and menopausal women for feeling and performing at their best: estrogen, progesterone, and testosterone. In balance, they make your body and mind run smoothly. When out of balance they can make you feel as if your world has been flipped upside down. This is why we encourage women in their midthirties, especially if you are already experiencing hormone-related symptoms, to begin testing, at minimum, for these three key hormones. It's a simple, relatively inexpensive hormone panel test, and it's covered by most insurance companies.

Why test? Because everything else is just a guess, right? The real reason we test women at the start of their midthirties is that this is when female fertility functions start slowing down. Women begin to experience changes in menstruation, such as changes in the frequency, length, discomfort, and blood flow of their cycles. They may also experience worsening PMS (migraines, food cravings, mood swings, and so forth) and other hormonal symptoms that suggest the onset of perimenopause, like drops in progesterone levels when they miss a menstrual month. This decline in progesterone relative to higher estrogen levels seems to be a common cause of PMS and perimenopausal and menopausal discomforts (Burger2008, 603–12; Desindes 2004, 2–4). Over time, an upset in the estrogen, progesterone, and testosterone balance can create a cascade of other hormonal disruptions in other glands and in the brain, which can result in a variety of other unpleasant, even scary, adverse symptoms.

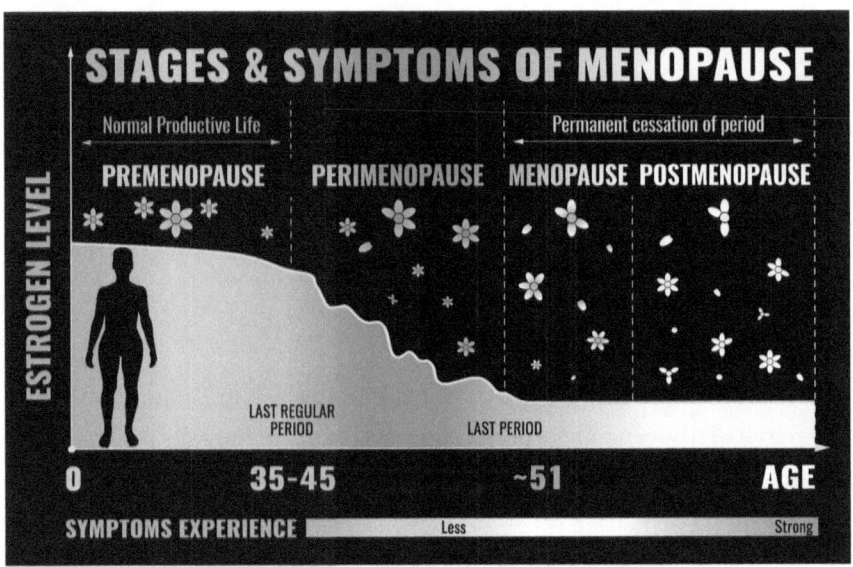

Feel free now to go back and review the symptoms list in this chapter associated with either too much or too little estrogen, progesterone, and testosterone. If you experience any of these, you should have your hormone levels tested. Then make sure your results conform with your symptoms. For all women, though, it is important to test and retest hormone levels. This way you and your women's health practitioner can work together to carefully monitor and correct any changes. In addition, you will want to create a comprehensive, customized holistic program that supports hormonal harmony.

Stop Counting Calories—Start Balancing Hormones

It is important to learn and understand that it's hormone messengers—not willpower or discovering the "miracle" fad diet—that triggers our bodies to burn fat. When our hormones are brought back to optimal levels, less willpower and less calorie counting are required. True health is found through hormonal balance, plus *consistently* eating, moving, and living in a healthier way. We promise that, when you find your health, you'll lose the weight.

Let's take a moment to talk about willpower—or lack of willpower and self-control. This is something we all struggle with at times—and need to an extent. See if you can relate to this scenario: You set out on a new low-calorie diet and see some weight loss within a week. You get really excited and feel good, but then around day ten to fourteen your hunger kicks in, energy plummets, and cravings intensify. Now, it's time to rely on finding the willpower to carry you through. The battle goes on until you give in to the cravings and hunger. You have had a setback, which slashes your perceived progress. You relied on willpower, and it failed you once again.

Unfortunately, almost all women can relate to this scenario. Although what most do not realize is that, when you diet, the hunger and craving signals you experience toward sweet, starchy, salty, fatty, "chocolatey" junk foods are not just "in your head." Researchers believe food cravings are caused by both psychological and physiological imbalances (Johnson and Kenny 2010, 635–641). Psychological cravings often are caused by our unresolved emotions and feelings. People may crave or abuse food and drink, either out of unconscious habit or addiction, or to cover up their lingering unpleasant emotions. The strongest physiological cravings often occur when the body or brain is deficient in certain essential elements. For instance, chocolate cravings are associated with having low levels of dopamine, our brain's "pleasure-seeking" neurotransmitter.

When you cut your calories too low, or remove whole food groups, you will probably experience psychological and physiological side effects. Hormone and chemical imbalances in your brain and nervous system will plague you with uncontrollable hunger and food cravings. In addition, sweet, starchy, salty, fatty foods are also considered highly palatable (for some more than others) and can elicit an addictive drug-like reaction in your brain and body, which further spoils your delicate hormonal balance.

You see, over many years of yo-yo dieting, poor food and sleep habits, stress, and limited activity, your hormones lose their potency due to the metabolic damage that is occurring inside your body. What does metabolic damage mean? It means your metabolism has shut down its normal hormonal activity. Hormones are either no longer relaying their chemical messages to other critical areas of the body, or the body no longer hears the messages clearly, or at all. It's similar to what happens when you smell something pungent as you first enter a room. Then, within minutes, you barely notice the smell. This same thing can happen when your hunger hormones are out of balance. Your brain no longer hears their messages of satiety and thinks you are starving. To adapt and respond as your metabolism slows, hunger signals increase, and cravings plague you. Over time, this cycle makes it nearly impossible to burn fat, and it wreaks havoc on all aspects of your well-being.

Help With 3 Key Hormones: Cortisol, Ghrelin, and Leptin

The B3H+ Program focuses on balancing three hunger hormones that are critical to you burning fat and reaching your own ideal, *healthy* weight. They are cortisol, ghrelin, and leptin. They directly communicate with your brain to monitor hunger, cravings, energy, metabolism, and satiety (fullness). Here is how they can affect your metabolism:

Cortisol, a "stress hormone," when working properly, is released from the adrenal glands (along with adrenaline) in response to a stressful situation (this is that old "fight or flight" mode). When this happens, sugar (aka glucose) is released into the blood, which in turn, gives us the energy we need to fight or flee the situation. This is a normal, healthy response to an acute bout of stress, which enables us to avoid danger and survive to fight another day. The process of moving intensely to avoid danger also releases other hormones like human growth hormone and testosterone, which help us repair damaged tissue, burn more energy from fat, and spare lean muscle. All this eventually sends feedback to the adrenal glands, and this suppresses the production of cortisol so we can go back to a calmer state ("rest and recover" mode). But the problems with cortisol begin when we are chronically stressed (whether we realize it or not), and do not offset its release of energy (glucose, aka sugar) with a burst of intense activity or other stress-lowering activity. The adrenal glands have to work harder during chronic stress, pumping out more cortisol, which eventually disrupts the production and levels of other hormones (leptin, insulin, progesterone, estrogen) and brain chemicals (serotonin, dopamine, GABA) (Tsigos et al. 2000). Also, when high amounts of cortisol are continually released and not immediately used for energy, the hormone acts negatively (along with insulin) as an unfriendly fat-storing, hunger-and-craving-creating, muscle-wasting hormone.

To positively influence cortisol levels, engage in stress-reducing activities such as meditation, breathing techniques, long walks in nature, laughing more, and getting quality sleep.

Ghrelin, a hunger stimulating hormone (which, when pronounced, even sounds like your stomach growling), is produced in the gut. Its job is to suppress hunger signals in response to the stomach stretching and the nutrient content of our digesting foods. With roots in the brain's hypothalamus (frontal lobe), this hormone tells the brain when you are either hungry or satiated. It's a kind of meal director, working on an hour-to-hour basis. Ghrelin levels rise when caloric intake is restricted, sending signals to the brain, telling us to eat more (Spears et al. 2011, 12). By stabilizing ghrelin levels, you free yourself from having to use iron-strength willpower to lose unwanted fat. The key to blunting ghrelin's hunger messages starts with slowing digestion in the gut.

To positively influence this hormone, try eating small amounts of quality proteins and adding fiber to all your meals. Plus, engage in short burst of higher intense exercise throughout the day.

Leptin, called the "satiety hormone," is made mostly in the fat cells and, like ghrelin, operates with the brain and our metabolic-stabilizing thyroid gland. When working well, it tells our brain we have enough energy (stored as fat) and shuts down hunger. It also sends signals to the thyroid gland instructing it to speed up the body's metabolism and release fat-burning hormones. This is your best case scenario! Unfortunately, if you become leptin resistant, from chronic overeating or under-eating, your brain and thyroid no longer get the message to stop eating and start burning. This is often why you see obese individuals eating as if they are starving. They have likely become leptin resistant. Note that very low leptin levels from chronic dieting and very high leptin levels from over-eating result in the same symptoms: increased hunger and suppressed metabolic rate (Barsh and Schwartz 2002, 589–600).

To positively influence the body's leptin levels, manage your stress, avoid prolonged periods of overeating and undereating, space meals out four to five hours apart, and eat your food slowly to support appropriate levels. Our B3H+ Program diet and our health experts can help you reactivate the body's response to leptin.

A Healthy Physical Environment—Creating Clarity and Wellness

All too often Western medicine is fixated on treating the symptoms and not the underlying causes or the individual. For this reason, B3H+ promotes a *preventive health* approach. We do this so you can make more of your own self-care decisions and take positive actions to slow the aging process and improve your body's natural healing systems. We are committed to shifting the trajectory of modern diseases. For example, our clients are challenged to question what they are putting in and on their bodies daily and what harmful things they may be exposed to in their environments. We want them to reduce their overall exposure to chemicals and toxins and to understand how they negatively affect their and their loved-ones' health.

According to Dana Suss, a B3H+ holistic health coach, the food industry is duping us by producing ingredient lists on their products that don't reflect the actual contents or potentially dangerous effects that may occur from exposure. Instead, they often list only what the manufacturer wants you to see, particularly in big, bold print on the front of the package.

This often misleads us into believing a product or food has your safety and health in mind. Unfortunately, this is rarely the case. And in fact, it's become so prevalent that the United States Pharmacopeia, a nonprofit group that sets standards used by the FDA, set up a database to track the infractions. It's called the Food Fraud Database. It describes food fraud as the "deliberate substitution, addition, tampering, or misrepresentation of food, food ingredients, or food packaging, or false or misleading statements made about a product for economic gain." It has a shocking number of entries.

You can bet that the wide and varied range of substances being added to our food sources as well as our beauty and household products cause disruptions in the endocrine system (the glands and tissues which produce hormones) and alter hormonal functions (Blum et al. 2015, 1862–1969; Sébédio 2017, 33–116). For example, eating too much (and a variety of) refined and processed sugar-fat foods in your diet can lead to insulin resistance. Insulin is a hormone released by your pancreas. Its major role is to signal tissues (muscle, liver, and fat cells) to take up blood glucose (sugar) to be used in the future for energy. These vital storage centers for glucose allow blood sugar levels to normalize. But, when you become insulin resistant, the receptors on these tissues, which normally allow uptake of glucose, no longer hear insulin's call to store. The result is chronically high levels of circulating blood glucose, which may eventually lead to type 2 diabetes, excess fat storage, and a whole host of other metabolic complications.

Or maybe you are unknowingly exposed to hormone-disrupting chemicals like bisphenol A (BPA), which is used to make certain plastics and resins. BPA is often found in the linings of metal food cans, plastic bottles, and storage containers. They have been shown to mimic or partially mimic hormones that occur naturally in the body, such as estrogen, and can interfere with hormonal function by potentially producing overstimulation (Alonso-Magdalena 2011, 201–207).

The good news is that you can avoid exposure to these endocrine disruptors and rebalance your hormonal health. Dana will support and facilitate your efforts by giving you steps to clear your homes of many hormone disruptors and by teaching you how to decipher what is potentially harmful in the products you are using and consuming. Check out more of her insightful perspectives in chapter 6, Holistic Health Coaching—An Essential Support.

How the B3H+ Program Worked for Me
Name: Christie
Age: 53
Starting weight: 207 pounds
Total weight lost: 21 pounds
Current weight: 186

When I scheduled my consultation at the B3H+ center, my main goals were weight loss and feeling better overall. I expected to get the typical diet with lots of salads and bland foods. I was shocked when I was told that I can eat many of the foods I love and still lose weight! Dr. Kealy's comprehensive blood panel test, Health 365, was the difference. It pinpointed the exact cause of my weight gain and isolated hormonal imbalances that made me feel … well, yucky! Who knew weight loss is not about how many calories you consume, but about balancing hormones that shape our appetite, hunger, and fat storage? And who knew that there is a very targeted blood test that gives you the information to help you get thin? I'm finally feeling optimistic and hopeful again about my weight issues and health. Thank God for Health 365!

Keeping a Positive Mental Environment

Dopamine

Weight gain can also be attributed to inadequate levels of dopamine, the pleasure-seeking and reward neurotransmitter released by the brain (Blum et al. 2015, 1862–1869). Dopamine deficiency can contribute to addictive behaviors such as stimulant use, overeating, drug and alcohol use, and compulsive shopping (Blum et al. 2015, 1862–1869). Without enough dopamine, your physical, as well as mental energy, can drop, making it impossible to concentrate. Next thing you know, you find yourself seeking out foods and substances like carbs, chocolate, and caffeine to keep your energy, memory, and focus going (Johnson and Kenny 2010, 635–641). When you eat whole foods that directly support and rebuild your brain's energy system, you will act and think clearer and will be more alert without the need for a "quick hit."

To positively influence your levels of dopamine, try drinking herbal teas throughout the day. Siberian ginseng and organic, decaffeinated green teas are great in the morning or midday and go a long way toward stabilizing energy and focus. Finally, a short bout of exercise can go a long way to boosting your dopamine levels, and it works instantly (Vučković 2010, 2777–2784). Simply climb a few flights of stairs or take a short walk to give you a natural jolt!

Dopamine and the Role of Genetics

Genetics plays a role in how dopamine—the pleasure-seeking neurotransmitter—works. "If you have the A1 variant (rs1800497) of the DRD2 dopamine receptor gene, which controls synthesis of dopamine D2 receptors, you'll have 30% to 40% fewer dopamine receptors, which can contribute to addiction risk, such as to food, alcohol, shopping or drugs," says Kenneth Blum, PhD, a neuroscientist who co-discovered this DRD2 addiction gene (aka "reward gene") variant in 1990. He works as a professor in the Department of Psychiatry at the McKnight Brain Institute at the

University of Florida. This addiction gene is present in about one-third of the United States population (a hundred million people!). The dopamine receptor gene variant actually blocks satiety and is one of hundreds of genes that behave in that way (McCulloch 2015, 26).

Hardwired to Eat 'n' Seek

This may seem odd to even suggest, but our distant ancestors' genes still play a role in our drive to eat sweet and fatty foods today. Around ten thousand years ago, in the prehistoric Betty Rubble era, calorie-dense foods high in fat and sugar (available only in fruits and the occasional beehive) were in great demand but were low in availability. The source of the next meal was all too often uncertain. Thus, our ancestors' genes evolved to hardwire them to prefer fatty foods and sweet treats. This genetically programmed behavior often made them gorge on sugar-fat foods when they were available in order to add to their fat stores. Extracting every scarce calorie and storing it efficiently as fat helped them survive the next famine, which could be caused by deep freeze, drought, or other circumstance (O'Rourke, 2014, 642–648).

Unfortunately, this legacy of our evolutionary past has geared modern man to seek out food often and hold onto calories to survive. This has become incredibly dangerous to our health, since most towns have an all-you-can-eat buffet. We are constantly surrounded by cheap, fast, nutrient-deficient, calorie-dense *faux* foods. We expend little to no energy gathering any of them because we buy them in twenty-four-hour stores. We are fattening ourselves meal by meal, day by day into "diabesity" (aka diabetes related to obesity) and sickness!

Here's the good news: Just because we are genetically hardwired to want to eat sugar-fat foods does not mean we cannot fight back and train our bodies to use our stockpiled fat for fuel. It won't always be easy, though, and a multifaceted approach is necessary to become an efficient fat burner. The B3H+ Program creates a metabolic spark so you can reignite your fat-burning machinery.

Other Causes of Hormonal Havoc as You Age

Other than the sex hormones (estrogen, progesterone, DHEA, and testosterone), thyroid hormones, and three hunger-regulating hormones (cortisol, ghrelin, and leptin) we have already highlighted, there are a handful of other hormones and factors that influence whether you will burn fat or store fat. They include insulin, "the friend of fat" (if chronically elevated); cholecystokinin (CCK), "an off-switch to hunger"; and human growth hormone, "the fountain of youth." This short list is certainly not all inclusive, but it gives you a picture of just how important your hormones are in the fat-loss formula. Other influencers include brain chemistry, outlook on life and health, social network, alcohol consumption, environmental toxins, sleep habits, gut health, movement practices, inflammation, stress (both perceived and actual stressors), and eating habits (quality and types of foods, frequency, quantity, and mindset while eating). These all impact your weight long term.

In other words, if your hormones are unbalanced and you have not begun to repair some of these underlying health issues and lifestyle habits, you are going to struggle more with all aspects of your health and wellness, in addition to your weight. This is *not* your fault, though, and most of all, *you are not a failure.* Rather, you are a complex, beautiful, resilient woman with many biochemical, physical, social, spiritual, and emotional components.

How Fat Flames Inflammation

Researchers suggest there are multiple ways in which our Western diet and lifestyle are causing adverse health problems, including excess weight gain and weight loss resistance (Newberry 2006, 1191–1205). One of the least-talked-about and biggest disruptors is systemic inflammation.

The fastest route to becoming inflamed is by storing an unhealthy amount of fat on your body. Particularly dangerous is excess fat around your belly. You see, the extra fat you carry does not just sit there; it is a highly active tissue. Your fat cells release a variety of chemical messengers, one of them being pro-inflammatory chemicals called cytokines. Cytokines are what your body uses to start the inflammatory process. For instance, you cut your hand while chopping vegetables for that healthy salad you eat every day now that you've changed your diet. The traumatized wound on your hand initiates an intense immune response that calls in a cascade of healing and protective chemicals like cytokines. The cytokines initiate the inflammation, which begins the natural healing process. The redness, pain, heat, and tenderness of the skin has to happen in order for you to heal swiftly and completely.

Similarly, when you are overweight or obese, your excess fat cells (releasing these inflammatory cytokines) cause low-grade, chronic, negative inflammatory responses (Monteiro et al. 2014, 20). All this fat-associated inflammation creates a host of harmful metabolic dysfunctions such as insulin resistance, appetite and satiety hormonal imbalances, lipidemia (painful swelling from excess fat), and rapid aging of tissues, making it nearly impossible to lose weight (Monteiro et al. 2014, 20). So, basically, all the extra fat you are carrying around, especially deep visceral belly fat (fat that gets stored in the abdomen around a number of important internal organs) is making you fatter! How is this even fair?

If you want to know if your body is inflamed, look honestly at yourself and ask, "How much excess fat do I carry around my middle?" Or, better yet, try a simple wall test: Stand facing a wall and walk in as close as you can get. If your belly prevents your toes from touching the wall, you are more at risk and likely to be suffering from some level of internal inflammation. This excess abdominal fat not only puts you at a higher risk for weight gain related to insulin resistance, but also inflammatory diseases such as atherosclerosis, cardiovascular disease, hypertension (high blood pressure), and cancer, among other things.

The best and fastest way to lower the inflammation and drop the pounds is to remove the sources of inflammation, like too much unmanaged stress (including the excess pounds) and let your body heal.

Hormone-Gut Connection
Your Digestive Fitness

In middle age, more than ever before, you will begin to see changes in your digestion. If you are exercising less and continuing to eat and to drink as you did when you were younger, you will more than likely begin experiencing digestive and intestinal distress. Symptoms may include fatigue, anxiety, food intolerances, allergies, "rock-gut" sensations, cravings, an "oil slick" in the toilet bowl from undigested fats, excessive bloating, cramping, gas, acid-reflux, weight gain, skin disruptions (rosacea, eczema), irregular (or lack of) bowel movements, and a general feeling of body pollution and ill health. Yikes! That is a lot to digest!

You may be wondering why these problems start. I will explain. The digestive system includes the mouth, esophagus, stomach, small and large intestines, plus the digestive organs: the pancreas, liver, gallbladder, and spleen. Most problems within the digestive system are created over time by our poor nutrition and a buildup of waste and toxins in the body. Under normal conditions, a healthy digestive system is an efficient assembly line that breaks down and processes food particles so that that food can be used as nourishment by our cells. Today our sluggish and distressed digestive systems are the root of many acute and chronic conditions, including a major cause of women's perimenopausal and menopausal symptoms.

The foods you eat, the way you combine them during a meal, and even the time you take to chew them thoroughly will either help or hinder the process. Everything you eat has to be broken down before it can pass through the walls of your intestines into your bloodstream to assist in synthesizing critical neurotransmitters (mood stabilizers, such as serotonin) in your brain, sex and metabolic hormones, muscle and connective tissues, nerve fibers, energy molecules, red blood cells, immune cells, and on and on. This process, in totality, is called *metabolism*.

You can probably start to see why less-than-stellar food choices actively breed poorer health and hormonal imbalances. Attaining a high level of digestive fitness is vital for you to fully absorb and assimilate the super powerful vitamins, minerals, and nutrients from the foods you eat.

Today, there is a plethora of research to support the connection between a healthy digestive system and your ability to lose the weight and to look and feel great. Below I introduce some of the benefits of maintaining a healthy gut, and I suggest an easy way for you to begin getting more of what you want out of the whole foods you consume. The list of major benefits include the following:

- Sustained energy and focus
- Balanced moods, less anxiety
- Happy and healthy gut bacteria
- Reduced sugary, starchy, fatty, salty food cravings
- Younger-looking, clearer skin
- Robust immunity, slowed aging process
- Weight loss
- Absorption of nutrients
- Optimal hormonal balance

There are essential substances that a youthful, healthy digestive system produces to enable you to break down your whole foods so you can attain and retain the benefits listed above. They are called digestive *enzymes*. These little proteins are responsible for you being able to induce biochemical changes in the foods you eat, so you can then produce new cells and substances that support building a better body. If your body is not properly digesting your food, you will suffer from a variety of negative symptoms.

Each digestive enzyme targets a single, specific substance to breakdown. Stomach enzymes include pepsin and betaine hydrochloric acid (HCL) that specifically target the digestion of proteins into amino acids, and help kill germs and harmful bacteria. Adequate HCL is also necessary to trigger the secretion of intestinal enzymes that help digest fats, carbohydrates, and other protein molecules (gluten, lectin, phytates). Intestinal enzymes include, but are not limited to, amylase (also released by salivary gland ducts, or tubes, in your mouth) to breakdown carbohydrates, lactase to break down lactose from dairy products, and lipase and bile to break down and separate fats into smaller droplets.

Besides a poor diet, two other key factors can affect your digestive fitness: aging and prolonged stress. Aging and prolonged stress both lower your stomach acid levels. Acid plays that essential role in breaking down food and signaling the release of other enzymes that further aid digestion. Chronic stress in particular is the most common reason, as it puts your body into fight-or-flight mode. When your body is constantly on "high alert," digestion is low on the priority scale, so it is dialed down. Thus, you will have impaired digestive enzyme production.

How do you know if you need digestive enzymes? One way is a stool sample test, which measures how well you are digesting your foods and if you are producing enough enzymes to break things down. If you would like to run one of these test, seek out a qualified integrative health practitioner.

If you are over thirty, experiencing digestive distress symptoms, or under chronic stress, you may consider doing a trial of digestive enzymes. It is the safest, easiest, and cheapest way to see if you notice any changes in your digestion. When you are ready, start with taking one high-quality digestive enzyme that targets all major food groups. Read the package label carefully and follow suggested doses. If you are unsure about reactions, dosage, and so forth, please talk with your healthcare provider. Taking one with each meal (or around the time you are eating) is a typical protocol. As you begin to heal your gut with dietary changes and begin to handle your stress better, you'll notice you will need them less and can try tapering your dose.

Also, please consider our proprietary blend of digestive enzymes to support optimal digestion. Our targeted delivery blend includes:

- **Dipeptidyl peptidase IV (DPPIV)**, a special enzyme that aids in the breakdown of gluten and casein, hard-to-digest proteins in wheat and milk.
- **Lactase**, the enzyme that digests lactose, known as "milk sugar"
- **Ox bile extract and lipase**, which helps emulsify and digest fats and fat-soluble vitamins

How the B3H+ Program Worked for Me

Name: Sharon

Age: 50

Starting weight: 191 pounds

Total weight lost: 52 pounds

Current weight: 139

I began the B3H+ Program in August of 2016. When I arrived, I had been suffering from terrible menstrual symptoms and was missing periods. I would often find myself keeling over with immense stomach pain and breaking out in cold sweats. My primary physician had put me on the pill to alleviate the pain. Not only was I opposed to taking pharmaceutical drugs that mask the symptoms, but the pill wreaked havoc on me emotionally.

Dr. Kealy, the Program's medical doctor, spent so much time with me reviewing various natural therapy options with favorable solutions. Her compassion and knowledge gave me renewed hope and confidence that I was in good hands. For the first time I was given a clear and basic, but thorough, understanding of what was happening inside me. Soon after I started the Program, my menstrual cramping subsided and my cycle normalized. Today, Dr. Kealy is working closely with me in restoring my hormonal imbalances and helping me stop the menopausal weight gain. Each week I learn new tips and tricks for how to eat and exercise for my unique metabolism, and how to keep my "hunger hormones" in check. As I age and my body changes, it's so wonderful to have a holistic doctor whom I trust helping me understand the links between hormones, aging, and weight loss.

At B3H+ centers, our medical team and women's health experts are actively teaching and sharing this vital information about hormones, digestion, health, and fat loss with women just like you. Women who may have felt like failures in their past attempts to lose weight are now discovering their best selves by naturally reactivating and rebalancing their metabolism and hormones.

Our program is designed to look holistically at your circumstances—your unique biochemical imbalances and other specific needs in the context of *your* life—to help you develop and sustain healthy eating and lifestyle habits, find and maintain your ideal target weight, and create a healing prescription for living. The result: A whole new you!

Now that you have a better understanding of how your body is changing and responding during this unpredictable but transformational period of life called menopause (or perimenopause), you are ready to delve further into the B3H+ Program. Let's discover how you can restore your health to lose the unwanted pounds.

References Chapter 3:

1. Alonso-Magdalena, P., et al., "Bisphenol-A Acts as a Potent Estrogen via Non-Classical Estrogen Triggered Pathways," *Molecular and Cellular Endocrinology* (2011); 355(2), 201-207.
2. Barsh, G. S., and Schwartz, M. W., "Genetic Approaches to Studying Energy Balance (perception and integration)," *Nature Reviews Genetics* (2002);3: 589–600.
3. Blum K., et al., "Clinically Combating Reward Deficiency Syndrome (RDS) with Dopamine Agonist Therapy as a Paradigm Shift: Dopamine for Dinner?" *Molecular Neurobiology* (2015);52(3):1862–1869.
4. Burger, H., et. al., "Cycle and Hormone Changes During Perimenopause: The key role of ovarian function," *Menopause* (New York, N.Y.) (2008); 15(4 Pt 1): 603–12.
5. Desindes, S., "Treatment of Vasomotor Symptoms During Perimenopause," *Menopause*: January/February (2004);Vol. 11(1):2-4.
6. Johnson, P., and P. Kenny, "Dopamine D2 Receptors in Addiction-like Reward Dysfunction and Compulsive Eating Obese Rats," *Nature Neuroscience* (2010); 13:635-641.

7. McCulloch, M., "Appetite Hormones." *Today's Dietician*. July 2015; Vol. 17(7):26.

8. Monteiro, R., et al., "Estrogen Signaling in Metabolic Inflammation," *Mediators of Inflammation* (2014); vol. 2014, Article ID 615917, 20 pages.

9. Newberry, E. P., et al., "Protection Against Western Diet–Induced Obesity and Hepatic Steatosis in Liver Fatty Acid–Binding Protein Knockout Mice," *Hepathology* (2006); Vol 44:1191–1205.

10. O'Rourke R. W., "Metabolic Thrift and the Genetic Basis of Human Obesity. Annals of Surgery," *Advanced Nutrition and Dietetics in Obesity* (2014);259(4): 642–648.

11. Sébédio J. L., "Metabolomics, Nutrition, and Potential Biomarkers of Food Quality, Intake, and Health Status." *Advances in Food and Nutrition Research* (2017);82:83–116.

12. Spears, A. C., et al., "Lifestyle Factors and Ghrelin: Critical review and implications for weight loss maintenance," *Obesity reviews: an official journal of the International Association for the Study of Obesity* (2011);12.

13. Tsigos, C., L. Kyrou, E. Kassi, et al., "Stress, Endocrine Physiology and Pathophysiology," [Updated 2016 Mar 10] In: De Groot, L. J., G. Chrousos, K. Dungan, et al., editors. Endotext [Internet]. South Dartmouth (MA): MDText. com, Inc. (2000).

14. Vučković, M.G., Q. Li, B. Fisher, et al., "Exercise Elevates Dopamine D2 Receptor in a Mouse Model of Parkinson's Disease: In Vivo Imaging with [^{18}F] Fallypride." *Movement Disorders* (2010);25(16):2777–2784.

CHAPTER 4
HOW THE BALANCE 3H+ PROGRAM SHEDS POUNDS

I n this chapter, we'll delve deeply into how the B3H+ Program works with your unique physiology. Don't worry, we won't get too "sciencey." The program replaces the old calories-in, calories-out model with the new science of hormonal balancing to naturally heal and boost your fat-burning physiology. We realize that balancing hormones may not sound sexy, but once you incorporate the fundamental nutritional and lifestyle changes, you'll transform the way you feel and see yourself during this midlife metamorphosis. In helping you find this optimal state of hormonal balance, you'll unlock your fat-burning potential. You accomplish this by placing focus on the basics of what goes into your body and what happens to it, from intake to elimination. Our program is designed to provide you with the principles and solutions you need for total health, fat loss, and longevity. Finally, our approach is sustainable and holistic. It integrates mind, body, and soul. It is uniquely designed to meet your mental, physical, and spiritual needs.

A Key Ingredient—Whole-Food Nutrition

Our bodies are reflections of what we eat, drink, and believe daily. They are like mirrors, showing us what is working well or—sadly—not working. What you choose to eat, drink, and believe can either sustain your health or pollute you from the inside out. Every meal is a new opportunity to build a more youthful body, heal, and create hormonal harmony. You will not find sustained health and vitality in pharmaceutical drugs, caffeine, sugar, artificial ingredients and colors, processed faux foods, and refined flours, many of which we can consider toxins. The first step is to remove these so-called foods and substances from your system to give your body a chance to rest. This is the only way to find out if they are contributing to your hidden causes of hormonal imbalances, inflammation, weight gain, or weight loss resistance. Don't worry, you can slowly reintroduce them after you've gone through the B3H+ Program to find out if you can handle them again.

A return to a real, earth-grown, whole-food nutritious diet is required. Sounds simple enough, but this recommendation can seem vague and confusing to some, thus is not always helpful. "Healthy" foods are often hard to recognize with the mass of offerings on the market shelves. In addition, some of these "health" foods may actually be stalling our weight loss efforts and making things worse. Plus, all too often, we ignore our body's feedback to the foods we are consuming. For instance, do you ever experience excessive bloating, gas, constipation, acid reflux, and fatigue after a meal?

These seemingly disconnected and transient symptoms are not normal after eating; neither are they part of getting older. They should be recognized as an allergic response or food sensitivity which engages the body's inflammatory cascade. You may be suffering from some low-level food intolerances (analogous to having an internal subclinical allergy) that leads to systemic inflammation, illness, hormonal havoc, and a sluggish metabolism. Through our integrative approach to diagnosis and treatment, our clients see a dramatic, lasting improvement in their food sensitivities and allergic responses without the use of drugs. We offer women an individualized solution for natural relief. You'll be surprised by how easy it is!

Food Elimination Resets Your Metabolism and Hormones

We're often asked, "Do I really have to eliminate certain food types to reset and repair my metabolism and hormones?" And every time, we answer the same: "Yes!" You must eliminate foods so you know how your body and mind are responding to what you are consuming. This helps us know how to specifically tailor an effective diet and lifestyle program for you.

Let's look at the top five, worst foods that may be sabotaging your health and contributing to your weight gain or weight-loss resistance. All of them may cause hormonal imbalances and digestive distress. They may compromise your immune system, promote fatigue, a foggy brain, and moodiness. Some may seem healthy to you but could be doing you more harm than good, adding years to your body and brain.

1. **Eliminating gluten** (not glorious). What is gluten? And why is it harmful? Gluten is a naturally occurring protein found mostly in varieties of wheat, rye, or barley grain. It is tough, sticky, and gluey (just as it sounds). When you eat gluten, it gradually forms mucus that coats your intestinal villi—those tiny fingers that project out from the wall of your intestines and work on absorbing nutrients from your food. After you consume gluten over years, it can build up like a plastic film on your gut wall and seriously interfere with the absorption of nutrients such as calcium, magnesium, vitamin D, and B12.

Several studies have suggested an association between gluten consumption and intestinal inflammation, changes in gut bacteria, gastrointestinal inflictions (such as abdominal pain, bloating, constipation, or diarrhea) and intestinal wall permeability, allowing gluten molecules and other food participles to enter the bloodstream (Biesiekierski et al. 2011, 508–514; Nijeboer et al. 2013, 435–440). This causes the immune system to think it's being invaded. It responds by increasing your level of inflammation; in other words, it initiates an autoimmune response. This is bad news! These insidious gastrointestinal problems vastly increase your chances of gaining weight and becoming more fat-loss resistant.

Gluten has also been linked to blood sugar instability, cravings, celiac disease, irritable bowel diseases, hormone imbalances, headaches, "brain fog," autoimmune disorders, and erosion of the myelin sheath (the fatty covering of every nerve in the body, including your brain and spinal cord), which eventually interrupts motor and sensory nerve pathways (Nijeboer et al. 2013, 435–440).

This long list of problems and the risk for future disorders makes gluten a top offender. Therefore, we recommend eliminating it from your diet for at least the first six weeks of the Program. I know it's hard, but we've found when our clients eliminate gluten-containing grains and the products that are seemingly gluten-free but have trace amounts (such as salad dressings, condiments, candy, ketchup, soy sauce, and deli meats), they experience a remarkable number of improvements in their health, energy, mood, and ability to lose weight.

If you cannot face giving up your gluten habit in one fell swoop, we can help you wean yourself off relatively painlessly and harmlessly with sprouted grain products. Sprouted grains have been allowed to sprout—or germinate—and then at the right moment, they are dried or kept wet to mix and make breads, pasta, muffins, and pastries. They are unrefined, whole seed products and are considered "flourless." They are sold frozen to preserve their nutritional benefits. Although they are not gluten free, they are lower in starch and contain a higher proportion of fiber and nutrients (vitamins and minerals) compared to their non-sprouted, "fortified," mass-produced compadres.

For more information about the adverse health effects of wheat and gluten, we recommend Dr. William Davis's book, *Wheat Belly: Lose the Wheat, Lose the Weight, and Find the Path Back to Health*. Dr. Davis is a world famous cardiologist and health crusader for a wheat-free, grain-free diet. His best-selling book shows how consuming modern-day foods that contain wheat are making us sick, fat, and fatigued. He also provides tips and recipes you can use to find your way back to optimal health.

2. **Swapping sugar with artificial sweeteners**. Sorry, ladies. Artificial sweeteners are not the solution. Short- and long-term use have been linked to a variety of uncomforting side effects like headaches, menstrual changes, bloating, cravings, weight gain, and more serious health problems like type 2 diabetes and brain chemical changes which depress our mood (Yang 2010, 101–108: Yeyi Zhu 2017; Huang et al. 2017, 614–622; Spencer 2016, 168–180). They've even been linked to cancer (Reuber 1978, 173–200). Another study suggests they contribute to raising insulin

and to compulsive eating patterns for some users (Qiao-Ping 2016, 75). I believe this myself, as I personally struggled to break a diet soda habit for years, and at times of extreme stress still have cravings for one. Ugh! This stuff is evil and highly addictive!

Our forty-eight-year-old client, Leslie, drank a small pot of coffee several times a day. She sweetened every cup with a packet of Splenda (sucralose-based sweetener). She had been gaining weight, experiencing strong food cravings, and overeating. She felt that Splenda was a good sugar substitute and a healthier choice. When we told Leslie to give up her caffeine to help her detox, she cried. So we agreed to keep her coffee consumption to just one small pot for another week, but to remove the artificial sweetener immediately. She happily agreed. Three days later, she contacted us and said she was feeling strong withdrawals to the artificial sweeteners and had no idea how addicted she had become. She went on for months wrestling with withdrawals and trying to satisfy her physical cravings. You may have noticed how your cravings for sweets and fatty foods and your weight have increased with your long-term use of artificial sweeteners. This is all too common, and studies confirm that this ironic fact occurs in both animals and human research trials (Swithers 2008, 161–173; Pierce 2007, 1969–1979).

A recent study in the *Yale Journal of Biology and Medicine* suggested artificial sweeteners in diet drinks cause a phenomenon called, "calorie dysregulation" (Yang Q 2010, 101–108). This occurs when the body loses its ability to correlate the degree of a food's sweetness to the its caloric load. This confuses your body's feedback system and teaches your body not to respond when you eat smaller amounts of calories from something super sweet. Your body loses its ability to sense how many calories you have taken in, so you become likely to ingest more sweets than you normally would. The takeaway point here is that sweetness without the calories ends up increasing your appetite and has you reaching for another piece of cake (Yang Q 2010, 101–108; Swithers 2008, 161–173). None of us can afford to make losing weight harder as we age or take on the health risk associated with using these chemicals.

Not to worry; there are a few sweeteners that you can experiment with fairly safely. They include:

- **Xylitol** is a natural compound that occurs in the body. Commercially it's made from sweet birch tree bark and is labeled a sugar alcohol. It tastes like sugar and has minimal effects on your metabolic hormones or blood sugar levels. It actually aids in building bones and muscle. In addition, xylitol has been shown to reduce tooth decay and can be found in natural toothpaste. Finally, xylitol helps make your body more alkaline, thus less acidic. The more alkaline you make your diet, the more likely you'll prevent or fight conditions like arthritis and cancer. The general theory behind balancing your pH is that some foods, such as grains, sugar, processed dairy, and large-scale factory-farmed meats, tend to increase the acidity of your blood, which is not good for you. Eating more fresh, "live" foods such as fresh fruits and vegetables makes your body more alkaline (closer to an ideal pH of 7 to 7.3 measured on a 14-point scale) and can protect against those conditions as well as shed pounds. Research also suggests that xylitol slows digestion or gastric emptying, which may help you feel more satisfied after a meal (Chukwuma 2015, 955-962). One point of caution, though: too high a consumption of sugar alcohol compounds, regardless of the fact that they are "natural," has been linked to digestive issues like gas, bloating, and loose stool (Mäkinen 2016, 131-142). Use this product conservatively at first to determine how your system tolerates sugar alcohols.

- **Raw organic honey** is a popular sweetener amongst health junkies as a favorable alternative to white refined sugar. It is the crude form immediately taken out of honeycomb cells. It contains vitamins, amino acids, enzymes, health boosting phytonutrients, and other natural elements that are completely void of refined sugar. Studies suggest raw organic honey can be used as a functional food in your diet because of the variety of health benefits it offers. Raw honey has been touted for helping lower triglycerides, preventing seasonal allergies (especially when you choose honey produced locally), improving sleep, and boosting the immune system (Larson-Meyer et al. 2010, 482–493). There is one big problem we see with substituting this healthier alternative: for some, natural honey elicits a similar insulin response as refined sugar and will raise blood sugar levels, which takes you out of fat-burning mode (Bahrami et al. 2009, 618–626). In addition, it can be a trigger food and a highly addictive substance. If you plan to use it, try combining the honey with cinnamon to lower its glucose-increasing effect, and use it sparingly. On the other hand, if you have a lot of weight to lose, are sensitive to concentrated carbohydrates, are struggling with sugar cravings or the blood sugar blues, you'll want to avoid it completely.

- **Stevia**, also known as the "candy leaf", comes from a plant native to Paraguay and Brazil. It is three hundred times sweeter than sugar, has zero calories, less than two carbohydrates per serving, and does not affect your metabolic fat-storing hormones. It can be purchased in both a liquid droplet form or as a powder. A little bit goes a long way, so use sparingly.

- **Truvia** is an all-natural sugar substitute made from a blend of sweeteners: erythritol (a fermented sugar alcohol) and stevia leaf extract. It contains zero calories, is less bitter than other natural sugar substitutes, and has little to no effect on blood sugar levels. It can be commonly found in gum, candy, and other products. Truvia also makes a baking blend that can be used to create sugar-free versions of your favorite sweet treats. Studies report no known side effects of using Truvia, unless extremely high doses are consumed in a single sitting on an empty stomach. Reported side effects include an upset stomach and loose stool. Again, use conservatively at first to determine how your system tolerates Truvia.

3. **Compensatory eating behaviors**. Do you ever decide to drastically restrict your calorie intake or even fast after a day of dietary indulgence?

These are called non-purging compensatory eating behaviors and are commonly practiced in order to prevent weight gain (Abebe et al. 2012, 32). They include behaviors such as the use of diet pills, excessive exercise, or dietary restraint (Abebe et al. 2012, 32). Compensatory eating behaviors may seem like a logical thing to do after a night out or a sugar-fat binge, but they often lead to disordered eating patterns, psychosocial problems (appearance satisfaction, self-concept, mood disorders), higher levels of eating and weight concerns, and physiological stress. Your best post-binge reset solution is to go immediately back to eating regular healthy meals three times a day. In order to quickly rebalance your blood sugar levels, hormones, and mood, your next meal needs to consist of a variety of fresh, whole, earth-given foods. Eating more high-fiber vegetables, lean proteins, and good fats (avocado, olive oil, coconut oil, nut butters, seeds) will enable you to gently return to the practice of nourishing yourself rather than continuing to punish your body, mind, and spirit.

4. **Filling up on fruit because it's natural.** The truth is, fruits can be your fat-loss friend or foe. It depends largely on how quickly your body converts a fruit into blood sugar. Thankfully, regardless of how quickly this conversion happens, fresh fruits are vitamin-packed foods and can be beneficial to your healthy lifestyle, although not always beneficial to your waistline. When you are seriously trying to retune your metabolism and get the scale to budge, there will be some you'll need to consume with caution. Thus, eating for fat loss and hormonal balance will not (for most of us; there are always exceptions) involve eating unlimited quantities of fruit. Particularly detrimental are the higher-glycemic (sugar) fruits which are the very sweet fruits, often lowest in fiber (your friendly blood sugar regulator). Theses super-sweet fruits promote large blood sugar surges that push you out of fat-burning mode and into sugar burning mode. Fruits such as bananas, dates, figs, pineapples, watermelons, mangos, and grapes are likely to lead to the vicious cycle of crashing and burning. In addition, these sweeter fruits create problems for people trying to lose weight by increasing appetite and carbohydrate cravings. Do your best to avoid eating the tropical fruits, as they are loaded with natural sugar and lowest in fiber.

As a general rule, the fat-burning or fat-storing potential of a food (such as fruit) can be determined by the ratio of sugar and starch to fiber. For instance, a banana contains between 17 and 31 grams of carbohydrates (depending on size) and only 3 wimpy grams of fiber, which translates into a relatively high number of calories coming from sugar vs. fibrous carbohydrates. In general, the more sugar you have, the less fiber you have, the more insulin and fat storage that food will create. This is not an ideal situation unless you are training hard like an athlete. Athletes' bodies can better handle the sugar surge, which helps with recovery, repair, and rebuilding muscle tissue.

This is important to remember and helpful to you in making better food choices. To optimize your weight, you'll want to focus on low-glycemic fruits that encourage fat burning and hormonal harmony. Favor tart and sour fruits like berry varieties, grapefruits, lemons, limes, and granny smith or crab apples. Also, do your best to buy organic and seasonal fruits to get more nutrients and limit your exposure to chemicals. These lower-glycemic fruits will become your go-to solutions if you want to feel less hungry, normalize your blood sugar, and enhance fat burning, not fat storage. If you eat fruits that are on the medium and high-glycemic list, that's fine, but then you must treat them as starches on your plate and limit your portions to keep you in an elevated fat-burning mode.

Low	Medium	High-glycemic
Blueberries	Apricots	Bananas
Raspberries	Avocados	Grapes
Strawberries	All melons except watermelon	Mangos
Blackberries	Nectarines and oranges	Papayas
Cherries	Peaches	Pineapples
Grapefruits	Plums	Watermelons
Lemons	Pomegranates	
Green Apples		

5. **Eliminating certain food groups: fats, carbohydrates, or proteins**.
The body gets its fuel to burn from three sources called macronutrients.

They are fats, carbohydrates (aka sugars), and proteins (aka amino acids). In order to get the best results and stimulate your body's fat-burning metabolism, you will need to experiment with your individual tolerance or response to each.

Today, more than ever before, it's essential to read food labels to gauge what's added to the packaged food products you are consuming. Also important is knowing the calories per serving size and total grams of protein, sugar, and fiber. Although the B3H+ Program does not endorse counting calories and spending hours balancing out your macronutrients, we do acknowledge that calories play a role in the weight loss equation—just not as much as we've been led to believe.

We emphasize that the types of foods you eat are more important than how much you eat. Why? Because when you eat enough high-quality foods, in the correct "balance" and in response to your body's biofeedback, you will be better able to control your appetite-regulating hormones and effortlessly reduce your overall caloric intake. What you eat stimulates a unique hormonal response. For instance, your relative macronutrient consumption (ratio between fat, carbs, and protein) at a meal determines the hormonal influence on metabolism. It determines whether you will burn fat or sugar for energy and whether you will decrease or increase ghrelin, cortisol, and insulin and balance leptin hormones. A healthy dietary approach adjusts the macronutrient intake to match your daily energy expenditure and requirements and goal weight. Plus, it balances the hormonal response during and after a meal. Hence, when your body is appropriately fed, it responds with optimal function and will be free of hunger, cravings, and energy swings for several hours after eating.

Let's examine each macronutrient and our bodies' responses to them.

Fats

In most cases, fat by itself is considered hormonally neutral. It does not stimulate the pancreas to release insulin (the fat-storing hormone) because it contains little to no glucose (sugar). So eating healthy, fattier foods (or fatty acids as they are biochemically known) plays an essential role in our entire body's function, particularly in the healthy production of hormones. The following foods are profoundly nourishing and help balance blood sugar: grass-fed meats; offal (organ meats); egg yolks; non-GMO, expeller-pressed oils; cold-water, low in mercury fatty fish (wild salmon, mahi mahi, sardines, and mackerel); and plants like olives, coconuts, nuts (but not peanuts), and seeds. (Note: GMO stands for genetically modified organisms.)

When we have a deficiency in our body's essential fatty nutrients, our bodies signal us to crave more fats. But often the kinds of fats we choose are junk foods that do not suppress our cravings or meet our nutritional needs. These junk foods typically pair low-quality fats with carbohydrates, which together have a detrimental effect on metabolism because they elevate fat-storing hormones. Thus, we put on weight as we become fat deficient. As you can see, cutting healthy fat sources out of your life is not the right approach to improving your eating and health.

Action Step: Get the Right Fat Balance for Your Body

Start by adding a healthy fat to each meal. Fat triggers the gut to release a hormone called cholecystokinin (CCK) and other gastrointestinal peptide hormones, which tell the brain that it's full. Also, add Omega 3 fats to your diet daily. Found in sources such as coconut, walnuts, and cold-water wild fish or high-quality fish supplement oils (or GLA—evening primrose oil) and algae oil (a good vegetarian and vegan option). Why? Because these fats help control how much fat is burned by the body and how fast it is burned. They also contain medium-chain fatty acids that help with weight loss and in manufacturing your hormones.

Sugary and Starchy Carbohydrates

You no longer have to look at the carbohydrate "issue" as black or white, or all or none. Your body can live without them if you choose to go cold turkey, but your emotions, hunger, cravings, and workouts may suffer. We have all probably experienced this after kicking starchy veggies, grains, sweets, and all fruit to the curb. We don't recommend this for most people, especially for women.

Finding their individual carbohydrate tolerance can be one of the most difficult challenges for our clients and often ends up being an on-going experiment. Don't worry, you won't have to carry a measuring cup when you go out to lunch with the girls. B3H+ helps you find your individualized carbohydrate balance, so you instinctively recognize your carbohydrate requirements without counting calories or obsessive measuring. This is unique for each person and his or her specific metabolism, as we all respond differently to sugary and starchy foods. Some are so sensitive to sugar and starch that no matter how much they eat, they have ill side effects, aside from storing excess fat. Others require a bit more to help stabilize their energy, appetite, and cravings. The most important thing to remember is that there is no one-size-fits-all approach.

Both scientific and anecdotal evidence suggests that most moderately healthy women, regardless of weight, feel and perform better when eating low to moderately-low amounts (somewhere between 50 to 150 grams per day) of carbohydrates, typically coming from a variety of high-fiber vegetables, nuts, and low-glycemic fruit (Hession et al. 2009, 36–50). This is true even as women transition into perimenopause and menopause and become more insulin resistant (more likely to store sugar as fat) due to the hormonal changes. The carbohydrate tolerance per person greatly depends on multiple factors, one being how much "gas" he or she needs to "drive" the car. For instance, highly active women often tell us they perform best and recover quicker on a slightly higher cyclical-carbohydrate diet, eating more carbs on the days they train hard, and fewer carbs on their off days. This makes a lot of sense and has support in the scientific community. Hence, if this is the case for highly active women, it would seem that less-active women need fewer carbohydrates. In general, this is true. Regardless of sex, most people benefit from eating a lower-carbohydrate diet and have better health markers to show for it.

Note that not just any carbohydrates will do, either. High-fiber, low-sugar, and low-starch carbs should make up the majority of your daily intake. This way you'll keep a steady supply of energy going to your brain, helping you feel satisfied, focused, and energetic for hours between meals. Remember, low-glycemic, high-quality foods digest slowly and are less likely to increase fat storage in the abdomen.

Always eat your carbohydrates with a protein, fibrous vegetable, and fat to slow its digestion rate. Also, add the acid from a fresh squeezed lemon or raw apple cider vinegar to lower its blood sugar response.

The key to finding your carbohydrate tolerance is in listening to your body's biofeedback after a meal, paying close attention to how you feel. Your body's whispers give you direct signals about what's working and what is not. If you don't experience hunger, cravings, or energy dips for four to six hours after a meal, you are likely eating in balance with your physiology and will be on your way to attaining your optimal weight. Yes, you read that correctly—four to six hours after a meal! Again, don't despair. We will help you zero in on a diet perfectly suited to you.

When shopping for carbohydrates, choose gluten-free, lower-glycemic, high-fiber carbs such as quinoa (our favorite because of the high protein content), soaked lentils, or black beans, millet, or sprouted buckwheat berries. Here are other examples of high fiber, slow-digesting carbs to experiment with.

High-Fiber, Slow-Digesting Carbohydrate Food List

Great northern beans	Steel-cut oats	Beets
Jicama	okra	Pumpkin
Wild grain rice	Edamame beans and pasta	
Squash (acorn, butternut, winter)		Plantains
Sweet potato/yams	Tomatoes	Chick peas
Navy beans	Turnips	Buckwheat

Action Step: Get Most of Your Carbs from Colorful, Fibrous Vegetables

Eat unlimited amounts of non-starchy vegetables for their antioxidants and satiety benefit.

Nonstarchy Vegetables Food List

Asparagus	Artichokes	Bean sprouts
Beet greens	Bell peppers	Broccoli
Brussel sprouts	Cabbage	Cauliflower
Celery	Chives	Dandelion greens
Green beans	Garlic	Kale
Swiss chard	Mushrooms	Mustard greens
Onion	Radishes	Spinach
Zucchini		

If you are eating other higher-carbohydrate veggies, beans, or gluten-free grains (meaning not from this nonstarchy veggie list) try to use them as condiments instead of part of the main course. Eat your protein, fat, and nonstarchy veggies first as they slow stomach emptying, which improves satiety too. They will keep your blood sugar stable and your insulin low so you can use stored fat as fuel.

Protein

Clean proteins pack a punch on our hormonal balance. Proteins are made from essential amino acids, which are the building blocks for healthy muscle, bone, hormones, and brain chemicals, which we need for mood and concentration. Protein plays a large role in regulating cravings and hunger. It aids in stimulating the pancreas to release a hormone called glucagon, which can help increase the use of fat for energy. Glucagon is required for maintaining muscle mass by shuttling amino acid building blocks and helps balance the effects of insulin, facilitating in fat loss (Schade et al. 1979, 874–886). Protein is also the second-most abundant substance in the body besides water. We need it for great hair, skin, nails, and to build and maintain muscle as we age so that we can become and stay leaner and firmer.

When we eat more protein in a meal than we do carbohydrates, we increase satiety, experience fewer cravings, and initiate the release of glucagon. The best sources of protein contain mostly protein, low to moderate amounts of naturally occurring fats, and very few carbohydrates, if any. They include all types of clean (antibiotic, hormone free) animal proteins; especially, grass fed bison and beef, free-range chicken and turkey, pasture-fed lamb and pork, game meats, wild cold-water fish, and shellfish.

Acceptable vegetarian and vegan proteins include hemp, nuts (not peanuts, which are legumes), egg whites and yolks, pea-rice protein, whey, grass-fed raw cheeses, and organic plain Greek yogurt. (Ova-lacto vegetarians may need to avoid dairy and eggs if experiencing inflammatory conditions or are fat-loss resistant.) It is absolutely essential for vegans and vegetarians to include a vegan protein powder in their diet to avoid the over consumption of grains and legumes, which can impact the immune system and hormones and can effect nutrient absorption.

Our B3H+ medical and nutritional team has developed a great-tasting non-GMO pea protein functional food shake powder. It is packed with 16 grams of high-quality protein per serving and offers a complete spectrum of all the amino acids you need, as well as your daily dose of essential vitamins and minerals. The vegan-friendly B3H+ Lean Body functional food protein powders come in two flavors, decadent chocolate and creamy vanilla, and are free of dairy, gluten, and soy. Each nutrient-rich food shake powder packet also contains eight grams of natural dietary fiber that provides satiety support, which helps control hunger. Check it out here: www.balance3hplus.com. We find this daily meal-replacement powder drink becomes a favorite and convenient meal option and enables clients to meet their nutritional requirements. Other vegetarian and vegan protein options may include rice, hemp, or nut powders. When choosing your protein sources, it is essential to read the label because vegetarian and vegan sources often contain a much higher proportion of sugar than protein.

Action Step: Choose Your Proteins Carefully

Eat small to moderate amounts of protein at most meals. If they are not free range, grass-fed (avoid corn, soy, and grain fed), hormone and antibiotic free, always choose a leaner cut of meat.

Why Diets Don't Work

Fad diets are everywhere. Maybe you have picked the latest one to go on. Most women turn to some combination of the "eat-less-and-exercise-more" approach. At the start you do just fine, and may actually lose a few pounds. You're thrilled. Being diligent and following a specific regimen has appeared to pay off. However, the female physiology is exquisitely sensitive to stress during menopause, and it registers this typical approach to dieting as stress. You start feeling hungrier, and your energy is less stable. You start getting cravings, and your metabolic rate declines. This is the body's normal protective mechanism and response. It's gone into starvation mode, so your body compensates by slowing your weight loss and stalling your metabolic rate. You may not understand this is happening, so you try harder, work out more, and eat less. You may see some more results, but you start feeling and experiencing other problems—things like gas, bloating, fatigue, sleeplessness, low libido, and irregular or disappearing menses. Guess what happens? You seek out advice and are told to eat more, exercise less. Reluctantly, you begin eating more. You gain weight fast and feel worse about yourself. You want answers. You seek them out again, but cannot find the right ones for you. So you go back to what you know: eat less, exercise more. The cycle and metabolic damage continues. This is why these diets are often referred to as "yo-yo diets." Frankly, this sample narrative is why most, if not all, fad diets don't work for people. This does not have to be you! We offer you a different, sane approach to achieving your weight loss goals and total health.

What recourse do you have? How do you begin to recover from the years of metabolic damage that's been created? Regardless of how your metabolic damage presents itself, you can repair your metabolism and never gain back the unwanted fat. Now is your time to take the first step in the journey toward attaining optimal health, hormone balance, and fat loss. The Program is designed to provide you with the specific tools and principles you'll need along the way. We educate you on everything you need to know about fixing your metabolism, rebalancing your hormones, and living younger, healthier, and happier longer.

The Program is based on the fact that there is a direct and indirect relationship between key hormones, body weight, and metabolism. The Program is a comprehensive, all-natural restorative health and fat-loss nutrition, supplement, and movement program. Our aim is to bring your body back into balance for newfound vitality and a juiciness for life. It's built upon the foundation of the following: Creating a personalized nutrition, supplement, and movement plan specific to your baseline hormone levels and other closely related blood test markers. We also take into account medical history, individual tendencies, and personal preferences. This information helps reveal exactly which types of foods and lifestyle program you will feel and perform best on. Plus, we also develop a customized master list of foods you should be eating more of in order to help orchestrate the hormonal and biochemical changes needed to reach your desirable fat loss goals. (We also give you a list of foods to avoid!)

How the Program Will Change Your Life

Here's what the program does:

1. Balances the three specific hunger hormones (cortisol, leptin, and ghrelin), balances the sex hormones, and boosts fat-burning hormones
2. Supports adrenal and thyroid health, and lowers systemic inflammation to boost metabolism, sex drive, and energy
3. Restores and maintains soft, supple, youthful-appearing skin
4. Returns a clear mind and more connected spirit
5. Prevents repeated weight gain and the yo-yo shuffle
6. Transforms the way you eat forever—the way you think about food, and your taste
7. Changes habits and cravings
8. Gives your body time to cleanse, heal, and recover from whatever affects foods and other stressors may be causing

9. Establishes healthy, restorative lifestyle practices: regular exercise, healing movements, journaling, sleep hygiene, personal growth
10. Empowers you to escape the suffering and stereotypes of menopause

Perimenopausal and menopausal women's wellness depends on maintaining nature's exquisite balance: a most delicate interplay of hormones and tissues that generate strength, stamina, overall vitality, sexual health, weight management, and a positive mental atmosphere. With this in mind, we offer you a variety of healthy—but tasty—meals, supplemental minerals, amino-acids and digestive enzymes, and gut-supporting prebiotics and probiotics. In addition, we recommend a daily vitamin supply to promote growth, health, and life itself, as well as regulate your appetite and metabolism. Our B3H+ Metabolic Weight-loss program is the first of its kind to holistically confront the challenges of the midlife transition and do it comprehensively and successfully for you.

B3H+ Program Process

First, you'll complete a Health 365 comprehensive blood test to help us identify which hormones may be out of balance and what to do about it. This is specifically tailored for women in their perimenopausal and menopausal stages of life. Our blood panel contains the following tests:

- Chemistry panel (complete metabolic panel with lipid)
- DHEA-S
- Estradiol
- Total estrogen
- Progesterone
- Pregnenolone
- Total and free testosterone
- TSH
- Free T3

- Free T4
- Cortisol
- Leptin

Next, you'll reboot and balance the hormones that are making you fat (cortisol, leptin, ghrelin, insulin, and so forth). Plus, you'll discover how to balance your hormones naturally so you can flourish in every aspect of your life.

You'll discover foods and lifestyle choices to reduce cravings for sugar, caffeine, dairy, fat, artificial sweeteners, and other foods that are not nutritionally beneficial. You will learn how your current eating habits may be contributing to your hormone issues and how to modify and improve your nutritional lifestyle choices.

Also, you'll learn how to create a positive mental atmosphere and embrace the sacred gift of perimenopause and menopause by tapping into the highly potent wisdom that accompanies this stage of life. You will gain a renewed sense of self-confidence as you take inspired action toward your goals. You'll learn empowering tools and new habits to rediscover what it's like to truly feel good about your body and your *self*.

Finally, you will have a knowledgeable, supportive, compassionate healthcare team, troubleshooting with you, guiding and empower you in your transformation and beyond.

Are you ready to begin your transformation? Nothing should limit you, so please don't limit yourself. You have a whole team by your side. We believe you can be better today, tomorrow, in your forties, fifties, sixties, and beyond—better than you've ever been in your whole life. We've seen it over and over again. As clients start to place their self-care at the top of their to-do list, things shift.

References Chapter 4:

1. Abebe, D. S., et al., "Binge Eating, Purging and Non-Purging Compensatory Behaviors Decreases from Adolescence to Adulthood. A Population Based Longitudinal Study," *BMC Public Health* (2012);12:32.

2. Bahrami M., et al., "Effects of Natural Honey Consumption in Diabetic Patients: An 8 Week Randomized Clinical Trial," *The International Journal of Food Sciences and Nutrition* (2009);60(7):618–26.

3. Biesiekierski, J. R., E. D. Newnham, et al., "Gluten Causes Gastrointestinal Symptoms in Subjects Without Celiac Disease: A Double-blind Randomized Placebo-controlled Trial," *The American Journal of Gastroenterology* (2011); 106:508–514.

4. Chukwuma, C.I., M.S. Islam, "Effects of Xylitol on Carbohydrate Digesting Enzymes Activity, Intestinal Glucose Absorption and Muscle Glucose Uptake: A Multi-mode Study," *Food & Function* (2015); 6(3):955–62.

5. Gaynor, Mitchell L., MD. 2016. *The Gene Therapy Plan: Taking Control of Your Destiny with Diet and Lifestyle.* New York: Viking Press.

6. Hession, M., et al., "Systematic Review of Randomized Controlled Trials of Low-Carbohydrate vs. Low-Fat/Low-Calorie Diets in the Management of Obesity and its Comorbidities," *Obesity Reviews* (2009);10:36–50.

7. Huang, M., et al., "Artificially Sweetened Beverages, Sugar-sweetened Beverages, Plain Water, and Incident Diabetes Mellitus in Postmenopausal Women: The Prospective Women's Health Initiative Observational Study," *The American Journal of Clinical Nutrition* (2017)106:(2) 614–622.

8. Iwasaki, S., et al., "Mechanism-based Pharmacokinetic/Pharmacodynamic Modeling of the Glucagon-like Peptide-1 Receptor Agonist Exenatide to Characterize its Anti-obesity Effects in Diet-induced Obese Mice.," *Journal of Pharmacology and Experimental Therapeutics* (2017);Vol. 362, 363.

9. Larson-Meyer, D. E., et al., "Effect of Honey Versus Sucrose on Appetite, Appetite-Regulating Hormones, and Postmeal Thermogenesis," *Journal of the American College of Nutrition* (2010); 29(5):482–93.

10. Mäkinen, K. K., "Gastrointestinal Disturbances Associated with the Consumption of Sugar Alcohols with Special Consideration of Xylitol: Scientific Review and Instructions for Dentists and Other Health-Care Professionals," *International Journal of Dentistry* (2016); Vol. 2016:131–142.

11. Nijeboer P., H. J. Bontkes, et al., "Non-celiac Gluten Sensitivity. Is it in The Gluten or The Grain?" *The Journal of Gastrointestinal and Liver Diseases* (2013); 22(4):435–40.

12. Pierce, W.D., et al., "Overeating by Young Obesity-prone and Lean Rats Caused by Tastes Associated with Low-Energy Foods," *Obesity* (2007); 15:1969–1979.

13. Qiao-Ping, Wang, et al., "Sucralose Promotes Food Intake through NPY and a Neuronal Fasting Response," *Cell Metabolism* (2016);24(1):75.

14. Reuber, M. D., "Carcinogenicity of Saccharin," *Environmental Health Perspectives* (1978); 25:173–200.

15. Schade, David S., et al., "The Role of Glucagon in the Regulation of Plasma Lipids," *Metabolism Clinical and Experimental* (1979);Vol. 28, 8:874–886.

16. Spencer, M., et al., "Artificial Sweeteners: A Systematic Review and Primer for Gastroenterologists," *Journal of Neurogastroenterology and Motility* (2016);22: 168–180.

17. Swithers, S. E., and T. L. Davidson, "A Role for Sweet Taste: Calorie Predictive Relations in Energy Regulation by Rats," *Behavioral Neuroscience* (2008); 122(1):161–173.

18. Yang Q., "Gain weight by "going diet? Artificial Sweeteners and The Neurobiology of Sugar Cravings: Neuroscience 2010." *The Yale Journal of Biology and Medicine* (2010);83(2):101–108.

19. Zhu, Yeyi, Sjurdur F. Olsen, et al., "Maternal Consumption of Artificially Sweetened Beverages During Pregnancy, and Offspring Growth Through 7 years of Age: A Prospective Cohort Study," *The International Journal of Epidemiology* (2017); 46(5):1499-1508.

CHAPTER 5
A METABOLIC APPROACH TO OPTIMAL HEALTH AND LASTING FAT LOSS

The B3H+ Program is the innovation of a team of weight-loss and hormone experts. Much of the Program's nutrition planning is managed by functional nutritionist, Jacqui Justice, M.S., C.N.S. She is a leading expert in fat-loss resistance, digestive wellness, and menopausal hormone issues. Jacqui brings over twenty years of experience to B3H+ centers. She has been featured in *The New York Times, Prevention, Redbook, Woman's Day, Organic Times, Westchester Magazine,* and *Serendipity,* and has been a guest health and nutrition expert on *Wake Up with Taylor* (Sirius), and the *Debbie Nigro Show* (WGCH Radio, New York). She also co-hosts the radio show, *It's Not Your Fault, It's Your Hormones* (WVOX Radio, New York). Named one of the top nutritionists in the New York area, Jacqui's first focus is always on testing and identifying the causes of hormonal imbalances and deficiencies associated with her clients' underlying health problems. She then designs individualized hormone-balancing nutrition and supplement plans for systemic healing and reducing body fat in specific areas of the body (for example, abdomen or hips). For instance, she offers eating strategies that address estrogen and progesterone imbalances; cortisol levels (high or low); thyroid support; menopause and polycystic ovarian syndrome (PCOS).

Jacqui, Dr. Siobhan Kealy, and other functional medicine practitioners collaborate to uncover what's causing our clients' premature aging, hormonal imbalances, ill health, and weight gain. Then they set out to repair and restore the body systems by balancing the hormone profiles once and for all. To do this, they perform comprehensive baseline and ongoing hormone and metabolic tests to check and monitor levels. They also conduct detailed symptom questionnaires to determine the specific nutrition and supplement plan required to switch the body's metabolism (for example, hormones) to achieve their desired results.

B3H+ Metabolic Weight-loss program: Three Phases

So now you are ready to begin the B3H+ eight-week program. Congratulations on making the commitment to living well longer. We are honored to be your supportive guides back to total health. You'll find the rewards are immense!

It consists of the following three phases.

Phase One (Step 1): B3H+ Metabolic Pre-Cleanse

The first step begins with the Metabolic Pre-Cleanse. This important step maximizes your success during the upcoming Fourteen-Day Metabolic Cleanse while helping you minimize uncomfortable detoxification symptoms. Many who have jumped head first into detoxifying can attest to experiencing stronger detoxification symptoms including headaches, fatigue, body aches, food cravings, belly bloat, "consti-poop-tion," or diarrhea. We find that women who ease into the Fourteen-Day Metabolic Cleanse, with five to seven days of the Metabolic Pre-Cleanse feel tremendously better during the full detox experience, with fewer crash-and-burn symptoms and more positive, longer-lasting results.

The first five to seven days of the Metabolic Pre-Cleanse is designed to re-energize you, reboot your metabolism, jumpstart your fat loss, and rebalance your body's alkalinity (creating a more neutral pH) so you can heal and prevent disease. The Metabolic Pre-Cleanse allows you to eat plenty of food. It entails eating three meals a day, with snacks in between, consisting of only real, whole foods. We provide you with a detailed list of approved and recommended foods that you can enjoy during the pre-cleanse process and throughout the entire program. You'll appreciate that the food we recommend tastes great and fills you up, unlike other diet foods that taste like twigs or leave you feeling light headed. During Phase 1, pre-cleansing, you will also begin to eliminate or limit the amount of processed and toxic non-foods and substances from your body. This phase can often be difficult, but by transitioning slowing and taking this simple first step, you ease your body into the Fourteen-Day Metabolic Cleanse.

Remember, even though we transition you slowly into the Fourteen-Day Metabolic Cleanse, you probably will experience some withdrawal symptoms and physical discomfort from pulling problem foods and chemical substances from your diet. Think of the pre-cleanse as similar to spring cleaning your home. During the cleaning, there is turmoil. So, when you feel some symptoms, like cravings or energy crashes, take heart! It means that the cleanse is working. Detoxification has begun.

Pre-cleansing opens the channels of elimination, especially in the liver and colon. Once the cleansing process begins, all the unhealthy toxins in your body get dislodged from the various tissues in which they've accumulated. It becomes especially important for the liver and colon to be ready to eliminate those newly dislodged toxins as efficiently as possible, as we don't want them lingering and making you feel worse.

There are a number of things you can do at this time to enhance toxic flushing and ease the body cleansing process. They include:

- **Drink, drink, and drink.** No, sorry we don't mean having a cocktail to get through the toughest moments of week one. We mean, drinking to stay hydrated throughout the day. As soon as you wake up, drink sixteen ounces of tepid or warm with fresh-squeezed lemon. Drink sixteen ounces of water no closer than thirty minutes before each meal and avoid drinking too much of anything during your meal to enhance digestive enzyme secretion. Drink water before bed, but not so much you find yourself waking to pee during the night. We don't want you to trade your good sleep for water intake. Aim for drinking half your body-weight in ounces per day, at minimum. Drink more if you live in a hot, humid environment or are exercising for long periods of time.

- **Eat every four to six hours.** Within an hour upon waking, start your day with a healthy meal containing foods (mostly veggies, healthy fat, and protein) from "My Weekly Grocery List" in the Appendix. Also, avoid eating or drinking anything but water, warm lemon water, or herbal tea two hours before bedtime. This has been shown to improve sleep and limit interference with critical fat-burning, muscle-building hormones (human growth hormone and testosterone) which are working hard for you at night (Salgado-Delgado et al. 2010, 1019–1029).

- **Fill up on fiber.** Fiber will satisfy your hunger, stabilize and lower your blood sugars during and after a meal, and streamline your digestion. Fill your shopping cart with dark-colored vegetables and high-fiber beans and fruits.

- **Heap up on healing foods.** During the pre-cleanse, you will eat well with three meals a day from the suggested foods list. With this being said, we want your plate to be loaded with only organic (ideally), once-living, nutrient-dense whole foods which contain a variety healing and detoxifying properties. (Go back and review the lists of high-fiber, slow-digesting carbohydrate foods and non-starchy vegetables in Chapter 4).

- **Eat organic.** Choosing organic foods whenever possible means you'll avoid a lot of toxic pesticides. If you are worried about the cost of buying exclusively organic produce, you can consider buying only the "dirty dozen" from the organic section, recommended on http://www.ewg.org:

Choose organic varieties of the "Dirty Dozen":

Celery	Snap peas	Cucumbers
Apples	Nectarines	Kale and all other greens
Tomatoes	Bell peppers	Potatoes
Berries	Spinach	Grapes

Safe-to-consume non-organic produce:

Onions	Sweet peas	Watermelon
Avocado	Asparagus	Grapefruit
Sweet corn	Kiwi	Sweet potato
Pineapple	Cabbage	Honeydew melon
Mangos	Eggplant	Cauliflower

- **Eliminate caffeine, alcohol, and nicotine.** These enemies of cleansing and detoxifying tax your adrenal glands and interfere with the liver's detoxification function. This creates more free radicals (unstable atoms that can damage cells and cause illness and aging) that your body will need to process later.

- **Alkalize your body.** A healthy body is a slightly alkalinized body. Meaning your blood's pH should be close to 7 (neutral/alkaline) on the 0 to 14 pH scale. When your pH is between 7 and 7.3, your cells and tissues will work properly, making you less susceptible to ill health and disease. On the other hand, an acidic body has been linked to joint inflammation, pain, gout, certain cancers, and other ill health conditions (Martinez-Zaguilan et al. 1996, 176–186; Kanbara et al. 2010, 45). Favoring specific alkalizing foods, such as plants and certain fruits, is the number-one way to alter how alkaline your body becomes. In addition to consuming more alkaline foods, try reducing the acid-forming foods in your diet, such as sugar, food additives and chemicals, fried foods, and drinks like coffee. Strive to make the majority of your meals alkaline based to help rebalance your body's pH. If you eat a more acid-based meal, make your next meal or two are alkaline forming. It's important to alkalinize your body to get the full detox benefits. If you need help getting an adequate amount of veggies into your diet, we have you covered. Try drinking our homemade pH Power Broth before breakfast, on an empty stomach, and then drink another one later in the day for a pick-me-up. It's a sure way to shift your body's pH from acid to alkaline.

As always, check with your functional medicine practitioner or health professional if you have a pre-existing condition, are pregnant, or taking prescription medications. You want to make sure that the timing and protocol of starting Phase 1, Pre–Cleansing is right for you.

Below is a simple quick start guide for Pre-Cleansing:

1. Drop the foods that are most likely to cause you weight gain, inflammation, and unbalanced blood sugar levels: All packaged foods, and any food containing gluten grains, peanuts, dairy products, white potatoes, sugar, alcohol, caffeine, artificial sweeteners, soy, corn, industrialized meats, and processed vegetable oils.

2. Eat three meals a day, with optional healthy snacks, from the Program guidebook of sample menus and suggested foods and snacks. Your B3H+ plate should typically consist of a variety of the following: high quality proteins such as shellfish; clean, grass-fed, pasture-raised meats; eggs (if tolerable); adequate amounts of healthy fats; non-starchy vegetables; high-fiber, low-glycemic carbohydrates; nuts (not peanuts, which are legumes and can be allergenic); seeds; and a variety of fresh herbs.

Phase One (Step 2): B3H+ Metabolic Cleanse

How long has it been since you felt truly great? Stop for a moment and take inventory of how you feel right now. Are you feeling tired, bloated, moody, flabby, achy, or spaced out? Do your clothes fit a little tighter than you might like? Are you suffering from allergies or food sensitivities? Are you so accustomed to feeling "off" that it seems routine? If so, let us show you how you can feel better in just fourteen days by paying attention to and changing what kinds of foods you eat, and more importantly, what you don't eat.

By now you realize the importance of a real, whole food source diet in the cleansing process, but that is only part of the total health formula. Getting to the root of health issues can be achieved by addressing a variety of controllable lifestyle factors, which we will continue to highlight throughout the book.

As you are learning, Phase 1 of the Program is all about eliminating the dietary clutter that is taxing your digestive and immune systems and slowing your metabolism. By eliminating the most common "trigger" foods, you can quickly determine which are working well with your biochemistry and which ones get in your way. The reward for doing this will be increased energy, improved focus, clearer skin, efficient digestion, hormonal balance, and a healthier muscle-to-fat ratio. Plus you'll likely release several pounds of waste and body fat!

Our Fourteen-Day Metabolic Cleanse is adapted from the nutritional and lifestyle guidelines that form the mainstay of our program. The cleanse, nutritional, and lifestyle guidelines work in agreement with each other to achieve and sustain hormonal harmony and total health.

We realize that, for most people, it's tough to choose healthy foods when your body is experiencing erratic hormonal fluctuations (ask any woman with unmanageable PMS cravings). There is a powerful action-reaction equation at work here. Weight gain, digestive issues, PMS, fatigue, mood swings, joint and muscle pain, and food sensitivities are just a handful of the many diet-related symptoms that can worsen with hormonal changes during middle age. Regardless of where you are on the symptom severity scale, the B3H+ Metabolic Cleanse will help alleviate your hormonal symptoms and end your battle with the midlife belly bulge.

The cleanse specifically focuses on naturally balancing your hormones—cortisol, leptin, ghrelin, insulin, and thyroid gland hormones—which, when in balance, boost your metabolism and burn fat. The cleanse also assists in reducing inflammation in the body by removing highly reactive foods from your diet like sugar, dairy, non-GMO soy and corn, vegetable oils, and trans fats. Inflammation is also reduced when fat loss occurs in the cleansing phase. When you have high levels of body fat, a poor diet, and imbalanced hormones you put your internal self in a state of chronic stress. If your body experiences long-term physiological stress, your immune system will kick into action and increase the release of pro-inflammatory chemicals. Chronic inflammation increases belly fat storage and dramatically increases our likelihood of becoming obese and insulin resistant (Huang et al. 2013, 86).

These pro-inflammatory chemicals may also mistakenly turn on your body's own tissues and begin attacking them as if they are foreign invaders and must be destroyed. This is an oversimplified highlight on how an autoimmune response or condition develops over time in the body. Our cleanse works to create the most favorable environment in the body to reduce common causes of inflammation, which lowers overall systemic stress and allows for fat burning to occur.

The Metabolic Cleanse is customized to support your hormonal balance by eliminating environmental and food toxins safely and effectively, all while decreasing and shrinking fat cells. It provides you with a natural and gentle release of the many toxins stored in your fat cells, liver, and colon. In addition, the B3H+ Metabolic Cleanse turns down the noise in your body and frees up your immune system to deal with other potentially more hazardous concerns like fighting off bad bacteria or viruses, accelerated aging, or out-of-control cell division. Regular cleansing is just good practice and is essential for living healthier and younger longer. Plus, it immediately goes to work to reignite an aging metabolism.

During the fourteen days, you will continue to eat real, whole foods (preferably organic) mainly from the Program's suggested food list (see the appendix). Although, instead of eating three healthy meals per day (like you did during the Pre-Cleanse week), you will begin to supplement two meals with our B3H+ Metabolic Cleanse whole food drink packets. If you get hungry between meals you can snack on healthy foods in moderation. However, before you snack, we will teach you how to tune into your body to make sure you are truly hungry and not just eating because you are bored, satisfying a habit, sleep deprived, and so forth.

Phase 1 also incorporates specifically targeted vitamins and supplements to enhance immunity and metabolic detoxification. For example, many of our clients have digestive problems and nutritional deficiencies. We offer supplemental support to heal and rebuild the health and effectiveness of the gastrointestinal tract's microbiota. We do this by incorporating prebiotics and probiotics, which act to support and rebalance the "good" bacteria living in the gut.

You Are Not Just What You Eat—You are What You Digest!

In addition to enhancing immune and liver function during Phase 1, we also work to rekindle your digestive fire. Our clients use our B3H+ Digestive Fitness supplement which contains a proprietary blend of enzymes, along with betaine HCL (hydrochloric acid, which triggers the release of enzymes) to support optimal digestion of fats, proteins, and carbohydrates. Enzymes are complex proteins which induce the breakdown of food substances into smaller, easy-to-digest particles. Each enzyme breaks down a specific substrate, either fat, protein, or carbohydrate. In order to fully absorb the nutrients from these food substances there must be adequate production of each specific digestive juice.

How Digestive Problems Start

As we age, we begin to experience a natural decline in these enzymes, which makes it difficult for our digestive system to effectively break down and absorb nutrients. Our enzyme production can also become sluggish and even inactive due to poor-quality dietary choices and an unbalanced lifestyle. It may be obvious there is a connection between bad eating habits and digestive health, but most people don't realize how chronic stress affects digestion. All stress places your body into a state of "fight or flight," a natural chemical response in the body designed to keep us alive. But, *chronic* and *unmanaged* lifestyle stressors—both real and perceived internal or extrinsic sources—may lead to insufficient production of stomach acid and natural enzymes in the body, interfering with our healthy digestive system (Taché 1989, 123-132; 2001, G173-G177).

Finally, you have probably heard the old phase, "tell me what you eat, and I'll tell you what you are." This nearly two-hundred-year-old statement comes to us courtesy of French food writer, Jean Anthelme Brillat-Savarin, author of *The Physiology of Taste*, published in 1825. While Jean's claim is true, we also have to include that you are what you *digest*, *assimilate*, and *absorb*. Therefore, you can be eating the highest-quality food in the world, but if more food is being ingested (as in overeating) than your body can efficiently use, digest, assimilate, and absorb into the bloodstream, you are overloading your entire system and are negatively altering the state of your health.

Hopefully, you can see the importance of properly managing diet and lifestyle stress in order to enhance your digestive function.

Do You Need Digestive Enzymes?

Particularly in the beginning of the Program, our clients require some digestive enzyme support. If you have the one or all of the following symptoms you'll likely also require some support from supplements:

- Bloating, burping, excessive gas after meals
- A surplus of abdominal fat
- A full feeling after eating only a small quantity of food
- Still feeling hungry or unsatisfied after a meal
- Frequent diarrhea or constipation
- Frequent indigestion or heartburn (components of undigested food bubbles back up into the esophagus)

Our B3H+® Digestive Fitness Proprietary Blend contains:

1. Betaine hydrochloride (HCL)—Helps in the production of stomach acid and the secretion of enzymes that assist in digesting fats, carbohydrates, and proteins

2.   Dipeptidyl peptidase IV (DPPIV)—A special enzyme that aids in the breakdown of gluten and casein (hard-to-digest proteins found in wheat and milk)
3.   Lactase—Helps to digest lactose, known as "milk sugar"
4.   Ox bile extract and lipase—Assists in digesting and emulsifying fats and fat-soluble vitamins

Recommended use: Take one capsule daily before meals or as recommended by the B3H+ medical doctor.

Now you are ready for Phase 2—The B3H+ Lean Body Weight Loss Plan.

Phase 2: Balance 3H+ Lean Body Plan

The Lean Body Plan is designed to support women's healthy fat loss and successful weight management while maintaining precious, age-defying lean muscle. It makes it easy for you to achieve the healthy weight loss results you want. It combines nourishing your body with hormone-balancing foods and our flavorful B3H+ functional food shakes. We also offer extra weight-loss-enhancing supplements, which are used twice daily to support natural hormone balance, fat loss, increased energy and satiety, and reduced cravings and internal stress. Clients always find Phase 2's protocol simple to follow and adaptable to their unique lifestyles, probably because we guide them the whole way. We'll do the same for you. Our mission is to ensure you understand how to best use the B3H+ weight loss support supplements and B3H+ functional food shakes, and that you are following the nourishing food plan for optimal success.

Our Fat Loss and Weight Management Philosophy

One of the keys to losing fat and keeping it off is maintaining muscle during weight loss. Why? Because muscle tissue is expensive to maintain, and it requires more calories to do this than body fat. For example, ten pounds of muscle may burn an additional fifty calories a day at rest, while ten pounds of fat burns close to twenty calories to maintain. Thus, the more lean muscle mass you maintain or build, the higher your overall metabolic rate will be (Elia 1999, 61–79).

On the contrary, when we start a restricted-calorie type of diet we lose fat mass, water weight, and some weight from muscle breakdown. When we lose our muscle mass, the metabolism compensates by slowing down, as it perceives the body is starving with a lower caloric intake. The metabolism is smart and creates a new, lower caloric set point for you to maintain to survive. This lowering of the metabolic set point is exactly what happens to people who yo-yo through calorie restricted diets, but later gain it all back. The metabolic set point is lower and running slower after restricted dieting, thus making it easy to pack on the pounds when you go back to old eating habits. Keeping your lean muscle will make it easier to lose fat and keep it off long term. It's the key to sustaining the lean and youthful body you desire. This is what the B3H+ Lean Body Plan is all about. In chapter 9, Fit and Fierce after Forty, you'll learn more about the Reboot fitness and restorative movement program, which works synergistically with Phase 2 in obtaining results.

Phase 2 gives you an opportunity to explore new and nourishing whole foods that are also incredibly effective for fat loss and muscle maintenance, as well as offering a plethora of other health longevity benefits. It is centered on eating readily available whole foods such as shellfish; grass-fed, pasture-raised meats; eggs; vegetables; fruits; seeds; nuts; and other unprocessed fat sources. Plus, it eliminates the most common inflammatory and metabolically taxing foods like gluten-containing grains and food products; dairy; non-GMO soy and corn; sugar; artificial sweeteners, colors, and flavorings; peanuts; processed oils and fats; and alcohol. Yes, sorry ladies, during Phases 1 and 2, we want you to pass on the alcohol (but not forever). A healthy liver is essential for metabolizing fat and processing toxins, which will help speed your fat loss, so for Phases 1 and 2, we want you to give your liver a rest. Plus, alcohol can cloud your judgment and make it easier to indulge.

The Lean Body Plan combines foods like those mentioned above with our high-protein, plant-based shakes and other nutrients to support your metabolism, maintain muscle, balance blood sugar, and control appetite and cravings. This comprehensive approach eliminates the all-too-common calorie-restricted dieting challenges and makes it easier for you to achieve and maintain healthy fat loss.

How the Lean Body Plan Works

It's simple! Replace two meals a day with the B3H+ Lean Body High-Fiber Protein Shakes, which can help restore your digestive system and repair the damage done by a standard American diet. Each shake contains 17 grams of non-GMO 100 percent premium pea protein, which helps control appetite and maintain muscle while you burn fat. You'll also eat one balanced, healthy meal on your own, sticking to the healthy food list (see the appendix). In addition, you have an optional snack each day to help stabilize blood sugars and prevent compensatory eating from occurring later on.

A nice thing about Phase 2 is that you do not have to spend hours each week buying or prepping in the kitchen for just one meal a day. You don't have to think about what to make for meals three times a day, which allows you to focus on other areas of work and life. We designed our program to be extremely convenient for you to incorporate into your busy schedules. We find most people choose either lunch or dinner as their daily meal. Having shakes for breakfast and lunch is most common because clients look forward to eating a healthy dinner each night and don't have to plan for meals during the day.

Your main meal of the day during Phase 2 should consist of unlimited amounts of nonstarchy vegetables; a source of clean protein (between 20 to 30 grams—four to six ounces of grilled salmon, chicken, or turkey) or a soy-and-gluten-free vegetarian choice; healthy fats (nuts, avocado, expeller-pressed olive oil, and so forth); and a small amount high-fiber, low-glycemic, slow-digesting carbs coming from nonvegetable sources. If you're hungry between meals, you can add any of the sample snacks below or create your own:

- Raw vegetables with two tablespoons of almond butter or home-made guacamole
- Half a cup of berries, a green salad with half an avocado and nuts or two tablespoons olive oil and lemon juice to taste
- Dried jerky (Go wild and create your own in a food dehydrator!)

B3H+ Weight Loss Support Packets

The B3H+ Weight Loss Support Supplement Packets are taken twice a day during Phase 2. Each packet contains a blend of the following:

- B3H+ Thermo (one capsule) is designed to support healthy weight loss by helping to increase the body's metabolic rate safely without causing any stimulant-associated side effects that are often found in other weight loss formulas.
- B3H+ Carnitine (2 capsules) is a comprehensive endocrine-and-metabolic-balancing formula designed to promote optimal body composition by favorably modulating the hormones insulin, leptin, and cortisol; balancing blood sugar; optimizing the lipoprotein lipase enzyme; and limiting cravings.
- B3H+ SkinnyTrim (two capsules) ingredients were chosen based on the latest research in overcoming the challenges of losing body fat while maintaining, and even increasing, lean body mass and basal metabolic rate. This formula is also designed to control appetite, the stress response, moods, and energy.

More Highlights of The B3H+ Lean Body Plan

- **Hormone levels testing:** We recommend all women over the age of forty get the Health 365 comprehensive blood panel test during Phase 2. This is typically completed by the end of week three in the program. The initial blood test results roughly indicate to our functional medicine doctors where your hormone levels are after a few weeks of gentle detoxification. We say roughly because the test may show adequate levels of a hormone, but your symptoms might indicate you need more. Regardless, the results of the test are critical and extremely useful in determining what specific hormones and nutrients should be targeted going forward in the program. The values we measure through blood testing are as follows:

- Leptin level
- Insulin level
- Cortisol level
- Hemoglobin A1C level
- Toxic metals levels
- Full lipid profile
- Particle-size panel, which checks for small and dense LDL particles that could potentially block arteries
- A full thyroid panel for things such as aging, obesity, hyper or hypothyroid disorders

Once the screening is completed, our doctors meet with you to discuss your results and provide you with a comprehensive medical report. Next, they develop a customized plan to naturally rebalance your hormones.

- **Nutritious physical activity:** One of the best things you can do to help boost your metabolism and maintain fat loss is to move more! Plus, physical activity is a simple way to continuing the detoxification process, via sweat, and it reduces stress within minutes. During Phase 2, we strongly encourage clients participate in, at minimum, a daily walking program. You have to start somewhere. So if you are new to exercise, brisk walking is a safe and fairly easy way to begin. All you need is a pair of comfy shoes and the willingness to carve out time in your day. Start by moving fifteen minutes per day. At the end of the first week, add another fifteen minutes to make it thirty minutes per day. Keep adding five to ten minutes each week till you are walking for an hour or more each day. Don't worry if you cannot get out for a full-hour session;

you can easily break it up into smaller sessions throughout the day. If you have already been working out, and are moving often, congratulations! Keep going, or consider bumping it up now. For more information on exercise and how it affects hormones and your health, turn now to chapter 9, Fit and Fierce after Forty. There you'll learn everything about our unique B3H+ Reboot Fitness Program and how our customized workouts are designed to spark your fat-burning hormones. We want you working out smarter with your body, not harder or against your body!

- **Journal it:** Why keep a journal? We believe it's critical to journal when you are starting your health paradigm shift. The more you can record the better. Keeping a detailed health journal chronicles things like your food intake, supplements, illnesses, allergies, exercise, water intake, and sleep habits. There are many advantages to keeping a detailed health journal:

  - It's one of the quickest ways to find out if what you are consuming is working for *you*. Plus, it allows you to notice any food sensitivities, intolerances, or allergies, which may be causing gas, bloating, joint pain, cramping, change in bowel habits, congestion, or skin reactions. When you have a history of your body's reactions to what you are eating, you can make adjustments sooner to improve symptoms.
  - Writing things down increases your likelihood of sticking to new habits and enables you to track progress. Dr. Gail Matthews, clinical psychologist and professor at Dominican University of California, reported that people who write down their goals and action steps for new health behavior have a 70 percent or higher success rate than their non-tracking peers. So, keep your journal close (or use an app on your smartphone), near your bed, office desk, or kitchen so you are reminded to write and stay on track.

- Writing things down enables you to see how lifestyle factors like sleep, stress levels, diet, hormones, and exercise habits are impacting your hunger, energy levels, and food cravings.

If you have never written in a journal before, we suggest doing it during Phase 1 and Phase 2. You'll be amazed at what you discover about your habits, food reactions, tendencies, and personal preferences.

Phase 3: The Balance 3H+ Whole Food Plan

The Whole Food Plan is the last phase of the Program. In Phase 3, you break the cleanse, phase out the lean body shakes, and reintegrate real, earth-gifted whole foods into your diet. Now is when you start preparing your own daily meals and snacks in order to continue the fat loss, healing, health, and detoxification benefits. We work closely with you to sustain your new-found energy, body composition changes, and feelings of well-being through specific menus, meal and snack ideas, and planning and food preparation techniques. We provide you with a recipe book filled with a variety of easy-to-prepare, nourishing, and tasty meal ideas, while staying with the proportions of the ideal meal. Clients find that most of our suggested recipes and cooking or preparation techniques work fairly effortlessly into their busy day-to-day life. We believe you will too.

Our nutritionists also provide direct guidance on what times are best to eat, so that you do not go more than four to six hours without food unless it is during an overnight fast. At night, after supper, is when you want your body to have a complete break from eating. Fasting each night (aka daily intermittent fasting) for a minimum of twelve to fourteen hours has been shown to enhance your body's ability to burn fat from areas that are inaccessible when in a fed state (Chen et al. 2016, 33739; Ferreira-Marques et al. 2016, 1470–1484; Ravussin et al. 2015, 1097–1104). Simply put, this occurs because your body gets a break from digesting and assimilating food (glucose and sugar) for energy. When your body does not have to use food for energy, it is forced to adapt and pull calories from the only source of energy available to it—the fat stored in your cells. Most folks enter a fasting state around twelve hours after their last meal. This is why twelve hours is the minimum time required to achieve the intermittent fasting benefits. Besides fat burning, there are other good reasons you'll want to experiment with extending your nightly fast. They include:

- Enhances cellular repair in tissues, reduces free radical damage (muscle, organs, and so forth) (Weindruch 1988; Masoro 1992, 1250S-1252S; Ravussin 2015, 1097–1104)
- Reduces risk for breast cancer in women (Cleary et al. 2002, 836–843; Chen et al. 2016, 33739)
- Can improve brain function and is neuroprotective (Ferreira-Marques et al. 2016, 1470–1484)
- Resets hunger hormones and insulin sensitivity (Halberg et al. 2005, 2128-2136; Ravussin et al. 2015, 1097–1104)
- Leads to a longer lifespan (Johnson 2007, 209–211; Ravussin et al. 2015, 1097–1104)

Here is an example of a simple fourteen-hour intermittent fasting schedule you could try: Don't eat between the hours of seven in the evening and nine in the morning. In other words, eat your first meal after nine o'clock in the morning and your last meal before seven o'clock each night.

Our food plans contain a few specifics, still avoiding high-problem, low-quality foods and nonfoods, and provides you with suggested sample menus for rebalancing your estrogen, progesterone, testosterone, insulin, thyroid, cortisol, leptin, and ghrelin. The food plans allows for some flexibility with useful parameters. Here's an example of a suggested menu for non-night-fasting days:

Breakfast—7:30 a.m.
8 ounces warm lemon water
3 to 4 ounces lean, clean protein; 1 low-glycemic fruit or vegetable; 1 healthy fat *(Example: – Leftover chicken sausage and stir-fried vegetables or pre-prepared vanilla chia pudding)*

Snack 1 (optional) —10:30 a.m.:
1 ounce lean, clean protein; 1 low-glycemic fruit or vegetable (if not eaten at breakfast) *(Examples: raw vegetables with hummus or 1 egg and ½ avocado)*

Lunch—12:30 p.m.:
4 ounces lean, clean protein or protein shake; 2+ servings of low-glycemic vegetables; 1 healthy fat *(Example: grilled chicken salad with olive oil and lemon juice)*

Snack 2 (optional) 3:30 p.m.:
1 ounce lean, clean protein, 1 low-glycemic fruit or vegetable *(Example: celery with 1 tablespoon almond butter)*

Dinner—7:30 p.m.:
4 ounces lean, clean protein or a B3H+ Functional Food, High Protein Shake, 1 serving complex starch; 2+ servings of low-glycemic vegetable, 1 healthy fat *(Example: salmon filet, grilled asparagus, ¼ sweet potato with cinnamon and ghee [clarified butter])*

In addition, you should consume ½ oz of water per pound of body weight per day, and more on exercise days.

Notice how the times are specific and that each meal is set up with a convenience option, like using last night's leftovers or pre-prepared meals as a preemptive eating strategy. Also notice that this type of plan establishes a strong routine to the eating strategy. Having a well-designed meal plan takes a lot of the guess work out of what and when to eat and will allow you more freedom in the long run.

With this being said, remember that the changes you have just made over the last several weeks are still new, so in the beginning you'll need to put more effort into shopping, planning, and preparing foods and meals. We promise that putting in the extra effort at the beginning will pay huge dividends. Plus, the last thing you want is to undo all the body healing and hormone balancing benefits by eating without thinking or planning.

In order to keep your post-cleanse glow, you'll want to completely avoid a diet filled with fried, heavy, or sugary-fatty foods. It is as important, if not more important, to do this final phase correctly as it is to do the cleanse/detox. It's critical to stick with eating meals that follow the B3H+ food plate (healthy fat, clean protein, loads of non-starchy vegetables, and smaller amounts of a higher-starch, higher-glycemic food, like beans and fruits). If you run into problems like food cravings, extreme hunger, or feeling deprived, or you find yourself slipping back into old eating patterns, write in your health journal to unveil what may be going on. Ask yourself: Are you really hungry? Are you filling up on foods for emotional reasons? Did you plan ahead of time to be sure you get enough of the right foods? Are you eating enough satiating foods like fat, clean protein, and fibrous veggies? Are you eating balanced meals every four to six hours or are you snacking all day, never reaching the point of real satisfaction?

The process of self-inquiry, self-honesty, and listening carefully to your body's internal cues and clues takes time to master and is often underappreciated because it requires you to slow way down. But it's invaluable if you want to change your habits for good. You must slow things down enough to notice why you are having these cravings and why you are overeating, skipping meals, and following other unhelpful habits. Slowing down in the beginning will ironically save you time and allow you to move faster with less thought and effort in the future.

Writing in your journal is a great way to slow things down and become more mindful about your feelings, beliefs, and thoughts about the food choices you are making during different times of the day, week, and month. Writing things down allows you to deal with the emotional aspects of long-held thinking and beliefs that impact your ability to make lasting changes with purpose, focus, and conscious choice.

You'll have days of weakness when you just want that dessert or "non-food" (insert your favorite indulgence here_____). Don't be too discouraged and beat yourself up. Everyone has these days. Don't try to compensate by skipping your next meal or by eating less the remainder of the day. This makes the bad hormonal situation created at your last meal even worse. Cutting back on the amount of foods (calories) you eat triggers hormones into action, resulting in unfavorable changes in your three hunger hormones: cortisol, ghrelin, and leptin. If you choose to do this, rather than changing the quality of foods you are eating, it won't be long before you break down and want to eat everything in sight.

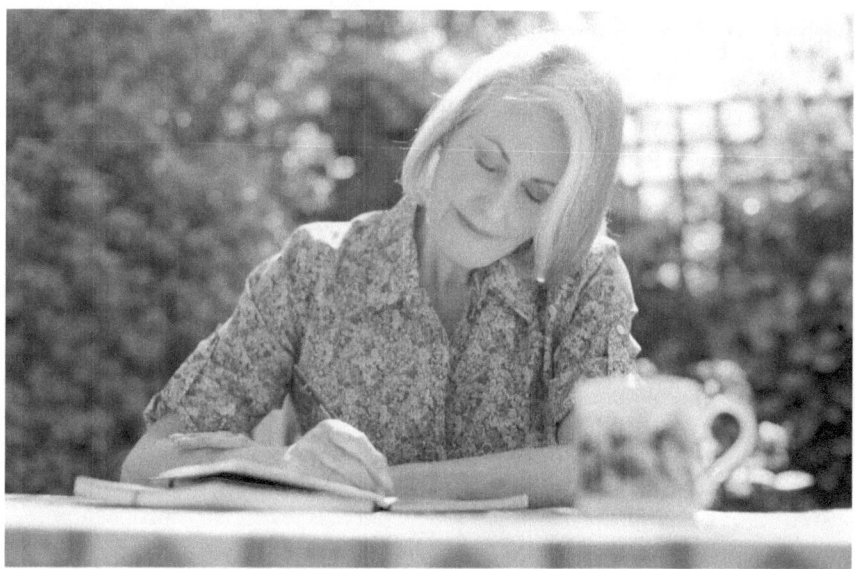

Another mistake we commonly see when clients hit bumps along the way is that they spiral into the usual broken-diet self-blame sessions, and they give in and eat more junk. The outer pressures or inner imbalances— or both—are at fault, not you or your intentions.

This is the time to just stop, become mindful, breathe deeply, and lengthen the exhales. Then begin to observe the emotions that surface, but with little attachment, as if they are just floating by. Next, look at what actually happened and determine how you can begin to rebalance yourself nutritionally, emotionally, physically, and spiritually. Write this in your journal now. Finally, write down the action steps you are going to commit to in order to rebalance and take good care of yourself. This simple self-care process is vital to getting you right back to your healthy eating plan and reconnecting with your reason for making these positive changes. You can move immediately into the direction of better health, hormonal balance, and fat loss at your very next meal. Just return to eating the foods that make you feel terrific. Before you know it, you'll feel better and will have saved yourself from self-defeating behaviors and guilt, uncomfortable symptoms, and potentially, ill health. Every one of us has setbacks when it comes to food and creating lasting lifestyle habits. But, with the right techniques, solid support system, and lots of practice (to make continuous progress, not perfection) we become gentler and kinder to ourselves when setbacks happen, and we can move past them more quickly and less painfully.

Final Words

Our clients primarily come to us for fat loss. They are sick of stubborn weight gain, and they don't know where it has come from. Seemingly overnight, they awakened in a body decades older than what they are used to, and they are frustrated by the lack of useful information out there specifically addressing perimenopausal and menopausal weight gain. They are tired of hearing the same old story: eat less, exercise more. Many feel hopeless as they learn the hard way just how often this approach fails. Then they visit us at Balance 3H Plus centers and embark on our integrative nutrition and hormone-balancing program, and they experience feelings of well-being within days. They have energy that they have not had in years, they are happier, sleeping better, are calmer, clearer in mind, and their joy and relief is visible in their faces. We hear comments like this one from our client, Tanya, who lost twelve pounds in twenty-eight days on the Program. She told us during a follow-up visit three months later, "I came in initially to achieve my optimal weight, but this program is so much more than that to me. I have no food cravings. I'm eating more regularly and continue to explore nutritional supplementation, and I do the occasional detox on my own successfully. I love the way I look, feel, and perform during my day! I'm a wife and mom, and I'm working full time. I've got a lot of my plate, but I'm so glad that I did the B3H+ Program." Every week we hear similar and just as powerful success stories from our clients. For us, hearing that our clients are living healthy, feeling amazing at any age, and loving their bodies again is, hands down, the most rewarding aspect of the Program for us.

It's your turn to be the best version of *you*. Allow this breakthrough medical weight loss and hormonal balancing program to help you get there. If you follow this integrative and functional, nature-based, 3-phase healing process, you'll experience amazing results. You'll rediscover a disease-resistant, energetic, and naturally healthy body.

References Chapter 5:

1. Chen, Y. et. al., "Effect of Intermittent Versus Chronic Calorie Restriction on Tumor Incidence: A Systematic Review and Meta-Analysis of Animal Studies." *Scientific Reports* (2016);6:33739.

2. Cleary M.P., et. al., "Weight-Cycling Decreases Incidence and Increases Latency of Mammary Tumors to a Greater Extent than does Chronic Caloric Restriction in Mouse Mammary Tumor Virus-transforming Growth Factor-Alpha Female Mice," *Cancer Epidemiology, Biomarkers & Prevention* (2002); 11(9):836–43.

3. Elia M., "Energy Metabolism: Tissue Determinants and Cellular Corollaries." In: Kinney, J. M., and H. N. Tucker, editors (1999. *Organ and Tissue Contribution to Metabolic Weight.* New York: Raven Press Ltd.

4. Ferreira-Marques, M. et al., "Caloric Restriction Stimulates Autophagy in Rat Cortical Neurons through Neuropeptide Y and Ghrelin Receptors Activation," *Aging* (Albany NY) 8.7 (2016):1470–1484.

5. Halberg N., et. al., "Effect of Intermittent Fasting and Refeeding on Insulin Action in Healthy Men." *Journal of Applied Physiology* (2005) Vol. 99(6): 2128-2136.

6. Huang, Jenq-Wen et al., "Metabolic Syndrome and Abdominal Fat Are Associated with Inflammation, but Not with Clinical Outcomes, in Peritoneal Dialysis Patients," *Cardiovascular Diabetology* 12 (2013):86.

7. Johnson, J. B. et. al., "The Effect on Health of Alternate Day Calorie Restriction: Eating Less and More than Needed on Alternate Days Prolongs Life," *Medical Hypotheses* (2007) Vol. 67(2):209 – 211.

8. Kanbara A, et al., "Urine Alkalization Facilitates Uric Acid Excretion," *Nutrition Journal* (2010);9:45.

9. Martinez-Zaguilan, R., et al., "Acidic pH Enhances the Invasive Behavior of Human Melanoma Cells," *Clinical & Experimental Metastasis* 14.2 (1996); 176–186.

10. Masoro, E. J. "Retardation of Aging Processes by Food Restriction: An Experimental Tool," *American Journal of Clinical Nutrition* (1992) vol. 55(6): 1250S–1252S.

11. Ravussin, E., et al., "A 2-Year Randomized Controlled Trial of Human Caloric Restriction: Feasibility and Effects on Predictors of Health Span and Longevity," *The journals of gerontology. Series A, Biological sciences and medical sciences* (2015) 70 (9):1097–1104.

12. Salgado-Delgado R. C., et. al., "Work or Food Intake During the Rest Phase Promotes Metabolic Disruption and Desynchrony of Liver Genes in Male Rats," *Endocrinology* (2010); 151(3):1019–1029.

13. Stawarz, K., et al., "Beyond Self-Tracking and Reminders: Designing Smartphone Apps That Support Habit Formation," In *Proceedings of the 33rd Annual ACM Conference on Human Factors in Computing Systems* (2015), ACM, New York, NY, USA, 2653–2662.

14. Taché Y. "Stress-Induced Alterations of Gastric Emptying." **Stress and Digestive Motility**, Eds. Bueno. L., S. Collins, J. L. Junien (John Libbey, Eurotext, Montrouge, France), (1989):123–132.

15. Taché, Y., et al., "Stress-Related Alterations of Gut Motor Function: Role of Brain Corticotropin-Releasing Factor Receptors," *American Journal of Physiology - Gastrointestinal and Liver Physiology*, Published 1, (2001);280(2): G173–G177.

16. Weindruch, R., and R. L. Walford, *The Retardation of Aging and Disease by Dietary Restriction*. Springfield: Thomas; 1988.

CHAPTER 6
HOLISTIC HEALTH COACHING

An Essential Support

At Balance 3H Plus centers, we always make sure that those who come to us receive all the health coaching and weight loss education they need along with their nutritional and hormonal therapies. We understand the value and importance of individual health coaching in balancing you emotionally as well as nutritionally. When you sign up for the Program, you will be assigned a dedicated health coach (aka a B3H+ Weight Loss Buddy) to achieve that balance. You may work with Dana Suss, Balance 3H Plus's resident health coach. Dana specializes in a holistic wellness approach, balancing the mind, body, and spirit to achieve desired, lasting results. She has extensive experience in stress management, sleep hygiene, nutrition coaching, detoxification, and women's health and hormones. Her focus is on healing the whole person and providing support while working through the Program. Dana is eager to help improve your physical and emotional health. She will give you the individualized attention you deserve. She creates a wellness strategy that works for you and helps you find the time to set up your new life—how to buy, prepare, and eat your food; exercise; reboot and relax—and still work and have a family and social life without added stress. With Dana, or any of our health coaches, by your side, you'll be better able to receive the benefits from the total program and achieve your wellness goals.

What Is A Health Coach?

As a health coach, Dana Suss is a wellness authority and supportive mentor who motivates and facilitates the integration of sustainable health changes into her clients' lives. She also helps clients cultivate a more loving and positive attitude about themselves, their bodies, and lives. Dana challenges clients to listen to their inner voices, identify their values, and transform their desires into actions. She gradually implements small changes at a manageable pace for each client. She teaches clients how to feel their best through food, movement, and other self-care behavior changes. Dana assists clients in discovering how each area of life affects health as a whole. Another focus for her is tailoring individualized wellness plans to meet a client's specific needs. For instance, she may design a wellness action plan to help clients feel their best by enhancing digestion, increasing energy, promoting hormonal balance, losing body fat, calming inflammation, and reducing or managing stress.

As a certified holistic health coach, Dana's core health philosophies and values include the following seven points:

1. True health cannot be achieved simply by eating more kale! While what you eat is definitely vital to fuel your body, Dana considers it "secondary" food. "Primary" food is more than what is on your plate. Primary food allows you to be your best self emotionally, physically, and spiritually. When you are fed with these, you can achieve your life's purpose. There is nothing more important than healthy, fulfilling relationships, nourishing movement, good sleep, having balance in your life, spiritual and restorative rituals, allowing yourself "putter time" (where you put yourself first and have no agenda), and anything else that speaks to your spirit and tops off your love cup. When "primary" food is balanced, your life feeds you, thus making what you eat seem "secondary."

In addition to traditional nutrition coaching, Dana facilities clients in identifying areas in their lives that require more "primary" nourishment.

2. Everybody and every *body*, is different! You may have heard the phrase "one person's nectar is another person's poison." Well, current research and even dietary guideline authorities are beginning to place more value on this idea. They recognize that there is no singular diet for optimal health or to prevent lifestyle-related diseases for everyone. This concept has been named bio-individuality. *Bio* means "life" in Greek, and *individuality* means "the particular character or aggregate of qualities that distinguish one person from others." This sounds like a mouthful, but bio-individuality is simply a theory that one key to health and happiness lies in recognizing and honoring our unique nutritional needs. For instance, a nutritious diet that works for one person may not work with someone else's physiology. Perhaps your partner lowers his carbohydrate intake and loses ten pounds in a week. You do the same and lose two pounds. Or maybe your girlfriend feels best fasting overnight until noon the next day. But when you try fasting for a week you get headaches and feel fatigued. See where we are going here? It's about finding what dietary program nourishes *you* and helps *you* reach your individual health goals.

After all, we are all as different on the inside as we look on the outside. Your genetics, health history, personal taste and preferences, age, blood type, metabolic rate, diet (the quantity and quality of what you consume), physical activity, stress levels, sleep habits, and exposure to toxins all influence your bio-individual needs. There is no one-size-fits-all diet, exercise plan, or lifestyle plan. Once you understand and accept this, you'll be able to integrate health habits that work uniquely into your lifestyle. You'll find that burning fat, keeping it off, and improving yourself becomes much easier because what you are eating is working *with* your physiology, not against it. The best person to understand what's best for you, is *you*!

3. Control stress—the root of most people's health issues! There will always be stress in life. Some stress you can control, and some that you can't. The amount of daily controllable and uncontrollable stress you are under is called your stress load. When your stress load is too heavy for too long, your body and well-being suffer. This unmanaged stress activates your sympathetic nervous system to initiate the "fight or flight" response raising cortisol, blood-sugar, and insulin, which creates inflammation. The inflammation reinforces insulin resistance and leptin resistance.

Remember, leptin is the hormone that regulates your sense of hunger and fullness. So, if you are resistant, you're likely to keep eating even after you're feeling full. The negative associations and sensations you feel when stressed are directly related to hormonal changes in motion. Rapid heart rate, increased blood pressure, muscle tension, digestive discomfort, and emotional upset from the lowering serotonin (a "feel good" neurotransmitter in your brain) and dopamine (a "pleasure" neurotransmitter in your brain that accompanies excitement) all manifest themselves in a particularly hormonal environment.

When this system is working overtime, you have a greater tendency to perceive everything in your environment as a possible threat to your survival. This "code red" response works to your advantage if you are, in fact, in a life-threatening situation; however, most of your modern-day stress will not likely kill you. All too often you end up with your stress button stuck in the "on" position. Dana strives to support clients in resetting their hormonal stress buttons by teaching them ways to manage stress using lifestyle hacks: optimizing sleep; eating healthy, nourishing foods; going to the gym to offset the high levels of stress hormones; practicing mind-body movements; journaling; meditating; and practicing breath work. Most importantly, she teaches clients how to make a conscious choice to accept stress as a part of life so that they can better anticipate and respond to it in a healthy way. When you're more mindful of health choices, thoughts, and habits, you control and manage the stress in your life better, rather than having it control you. If you are living the B3H+ lifestyle, each of your daily stressors will be perceived as less of a threat. When stress has less of a negative effect on your body and mind, then restoring your health, hormones, and metabolism becomes much easier.

4. The body wants to heal! Your body's ability to heal is greater than most believe. Without conscious involvement or awareness on your part, your body's cells know exactly when to grow and when to turn off, and when to repair and heal your damaged tissues and systems. Everyday damaged and dead cells are replaced in enormous numbers in our blood, skin, gut, and mouth. You could not stop this astonishing self-healing process if you wanted to; your cells do this automatically. The body's healing potential is so powerful. Its innate wisdom is always working the biochemistry and energetic transformations required to restore and maintain balance within. It's a beautiful gift when well taken care of.

If this is true, then why aren't we healing and in better health? The answer is that we erect barriers to our own healing. We often "treat" our symptoms as the illness, when they are often messengers from our body asking for help. This "treatment" of the disease symptoms makes the situation worse. A good example is high blood pressure (HBP). One of the causes of HBP is sticky, thick, sluggish blood (due to dehydration, smoking, sleep apnea, some diseases, and lack of healthy nourishing dietary fats), which restricts blood's free-flowing movement through the smaller capillaries. When the blood is sticky and thick, the red blood cells are more prone to clumping together. So, the heart works harder to ensure the clumped blood still circulates out to the smaller vessels, thereby raising blood pressure. This is your body's way of ensuring your thick, oxygen carrying blood reaches all your cells. If it does not do this, cells will die due to lack of oxygen and nutrients. What's even worse is that conventional medicine treats HBP as the disease, ordering medicines to artificially lower the pressure the heart encounters when pumping out blood. Although that may be helpful in some cases, treating HBP alone, and not the thickening blood issue, leaves the cause unresolved. The cause of the thickening blood must be addressed in order to normalize the blood pressure.

In order to reactivate and restore your body's innate healing potential, you must embrace it, learn to hear what it is really asking for, then avoid and remove blocks which interfere with it or shut it down (for example, the use of artificial chemicals, sugar, or drugs). Dana will show you techniques that can connect you to your body's inner wisdom, to recognize what it is "telling you," thereby removing the blocks which hold your healing potential prisoner.

5. Your genes are not your destiny! Each of us has a variety of unique features and traits that are written by our individual genes. We used to think our genetic makeup (DNA) was inked-in like a script that never changes, but current research suggests that this script can be produced (modified) differently through our environmental exposures. This is the study of *epigenetics*, which means "in addition to changes in genetic sequence" or more specifically, "additional information layered on top of the sequence of letters (strings of molecules, A, C, G and T) that makes up DNA" (Waddington 1942, 18–20). What does this mean? How does it relate to you and your health? Basically, any outside influences that can be detected by the body have the potential to cause epigenetic modifications. Therefore, your nongenetic exposures become the primary driver of health and disease. In fact, the choices you make in your lifetime predict 90 percent of your disease risk and early death (Willett 2002, 695–698). Nongenetic variables contributing to the risk for disease include things such as your behaviors, diet, air and water quality, social interactions, parent's health during conception, and other environmental exposures. All of these potentially drive epigenetic processes, thus altering your gene expression and the development of disease and ill-health (Willett 2002, 695–698).

A well-characterized example is Bisphenol A (BPA), an additive which has been used to make plastic bottles, food can linings, and store receipt paper. It has been linked to cancer and other diseases. Research suggests BPA exerts its toxic effects on our health (particularly our thyroid gland) through a number of different mechanisms, including epigenetic modification (Singh 2012, 10143–10153).

Furthermore, through epigenetic inheritance, some of the experiences from your parents can be passed onto you (Heard 2014, 95–109). At the same time, this epigenome remains flexible as your environmental conditions continue to change. For example, you may have inherited a breast cancer gene called BRCA1. Having the gene may make you more susceptible to developing breast cancer, but your lifestyle behaviors and environmental conditions will heavily influence whether it's "switched on." This means that, by changing environmental conditions, you can avoid or reverse health conditions for which you hold a genetic predisposition. They are *not your fate*. Having this knowledge is extremely empowering. You now know that you *do* have the means to take complete control of your health destiny. Your lifestyle choices influence the presentation of diseases you may be genetically at risk for. The reins of your health are in your own hands.

6. Treat the root cause, the person, not just symptoms! Conventional (modern) medical doctors are well trained to treat and suppress their patient's symptoms and help them avoid disability and death by disease. Often this is accomplished through modern medical treatments and the use of pharmaceuticals. According to www.infoplease.com, in the last fifty years, these advanced treatments and drugs have significantly increased the average life expectancy for both sexes (from 69.7 years in 1960 to around 78 years in 2010) and lowered death rates from various lifestyle related diseases. Despite these gains and improvements, mainstream medicine's persistent focus on quickly prescribing conventional tests, drugs, and procedures to improve patients' symptoms are not considered a viable long-term solution by the majority of functional medical practitioners. Treating the symptoms only, but not paying attention to patients' health and lifestyle habits and tendencies, does nothing to improve self-care, health longevity, and disease prevention. As a result, the underlying causes of the diseased state are not identified. Patients receive little or no benefit, fail to learn lifestyle changes that would improve their conditions, and often feel hopeless or worse about ever healing.

When there is an imbalance in the system, your body sends you signals in the form of symptoms. When symptoms are present, Dana and our functional medical experts probe more deeply to discover the source of the condition. Let's use the persistent migraine example. You come into Dana's office and share that you have debilitating migraines. Dana requests a dietary history log and discovers that you are eating dairy products daily. She knows dairy consumption, be it milk, cheese or yogurt, can potentially trigger food allergy reactions, in this case a migraine. She would work closely with you to shift dairy out of your diet for a while to see if you respond well and are free of migraines.

7. Follow these tips to bounce back after a "splurge surge." Despite our best intentions, it's easy to overeat or have an occasional emotional binge eating session. We have all been there! Whether it is reaching out for another chili cheese French fry even after we feel full, or eating an entire carton of chocolate ice cream during PMS week, suddenly you are stuffed like a turkey, feeling guilty and ashamed that you weren't paying "full" (pun intended) attention while you ate. Don't panic. We all have unplanned slipups and setbacks in life, especially with our diets. It's part of being an imperfect human in the modern world, working to make healthy food choices. Getting yourself back to eating well again after a binge can be tricky.

Check out Dana's action steps to help you recover safely and reset quickly:

- Start and end your day with an alkalizing cup of hot, fresh-squeezed lemon water. Drinking hot lemon water aids in digestion by stimulating stomach digestive enzymes, plus the vitamin C in lemons helps the body absorb more minerals from your real food diet. The fruit also contains an antioxidant called d-lemonene, which helps to flush out compounds present in the liver that are toxic to cells. In order to rebound quickly from going whole-hog over the weekend, plan to drink multiple glasses of hot lemon water the next day.

- Stay hydrated throughout the day. Yes, we covered this in chapter 4, but the importance of adequate hydration cannot be overemphasized. So why is it so important to hydrate the day after eating foods high in fat, sugar, and salt (or any day, for that matter)? If you remain dehydrated your body has no way of flushing out the toxins. Therefore, in an effort to protect your vital organs, your body will store toxins in fat tissue. Over time, these pollutants in your fat tissue are released, which disrupts normal thyroid function and hormonal balance. Dana's hydration action step: Aim for drinking half your bodyweight in ounces of water per day. For instance, if you weigh 150 pounds (68 kilograms) you should strive to drink 75 ounces a day. Also, don't forget to adjust for your activity level. The American College of Sports Medicine recommends adding twelve ounces of water to your daily total for every thirty minutes that you workout.

- Get out and move! Nothing works better than a hot, sweaty, metabolism-boosting exercise session to enhance detoxification and calorie usage for hours or even days after you've over indulged. The two types of exercise that work best are both "burst-style" exercise, sometimes called interval training. The first one: Sprint or jog for thirty seconds and then do a "recovery walk" for two minutes. Repeat this four to eight times. The second one: Lift the heaviest weight you can *safely* handle with near perfect form, and then rest for just under one minute. Immediately move onto a new exercise. Repeat this circuit several times. Focus on body weight, free-weight, and cable-system exercises rather than machines. This higher-intensity exercise raises lactic acid, which in turn elevates fat burning and muscle building hormones, which all are responsible for the increased caloric after-burn effect. If, for any reason, a high-intensity workout is not your thing or not safe for you, no worries. Any type of rhythmic, full-body movement will benefit you. Activities such as walking, biking, running, rollerblading, swimming, Zumba, yoga, or Pilates all produce positive detoxification effects. Everything—your cognitive function, stress levels, heart, lunges, joint flexibility, stomach, vascular system—feels rejuvenated and cleansed through exercise.

- Sweat it out in a Finnish or infrared sauna (nontoxic and low–electromagnetic field [EMF] infrared saunas are best). Both types of sauna can significantly expedite the detoxification process by heating your core body temperature, which encourages a deep sweat that makes the heart beat faster; increases blood flow, which lowers blood pressure; and allows your body to recover quicker. Saunas may also aid in calming inflammation and in healing joint and muscle tissues.

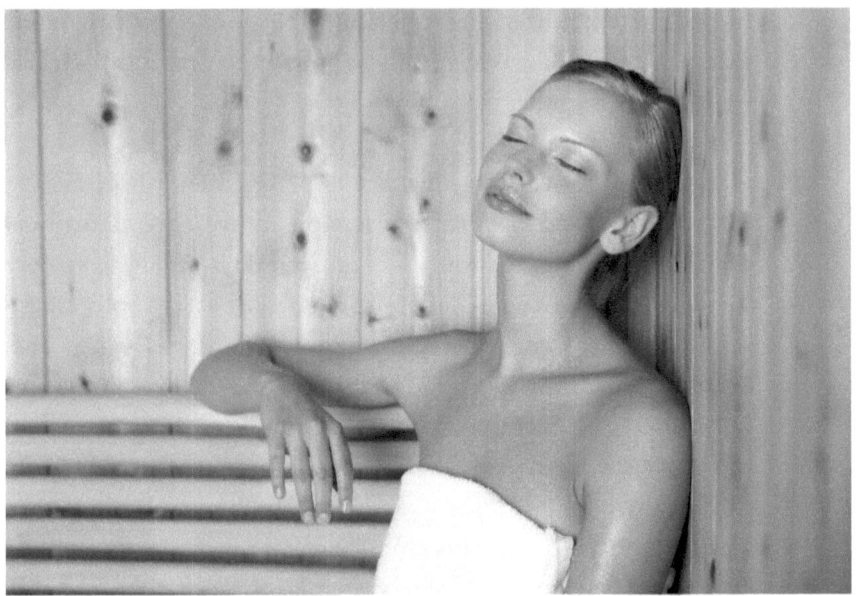

- Your body will forgive you, so start forgiving yourself! There will always be particular pitfalls that you know are going to be tough to survive unscathed: holiday parties, family dinners, buffet restaurants, or a weekend in Las Vegas at an all-inclusive resort with friends. These kinds of things are never total surprises; you pretty much know they are going to happen at some time. And when they do, the last thing you want to create in your body after overindulging is more internal stress. Give yourself permission to be perfectly imperfect. Give yourself some freedom to fail, so that when you "think" you did, you will not dwell on it. Remember that life is full of momentary setbacks. Your health success should be measured less by the percentage of time you stay on your eating plan, and more on how gracefully you handle the disappointment and effectively overcome setbacks. There is no need fall prey to negative thinking and defeating self-talk. This only drains you of energy and keeps you from living your true purpose and sharing your unique gifts with the world. In addition to changing the tone of your thoughts and learning to forgive yourself, you can do things that make you better prepared to avoid most of these setbacks. Some clients like to keep a stash of jerky, raw nuts, and apples on hand. This way, when (not if) they find themselves in a "food conundrum," they are set no matter what happens or where they are in the day. By planning ahead and keeping your pantry, purse, and car well stocked, you'll worry less about overeating the wrong foods for your body.

Final Words

Instead of stressing or gritting your way through perimenopause and menopause, try practicing an attitude of gratitude. I know what you are thinking—this sounds too "woo-woo" for me. But it does produce real change if you practice gratitude daily. Dana strongly advocates that you become a *gratitudarian*—a person who can be thankful for today and all that it brings. No regrets, just lessons. Less stress, more acceptance. Fewer expectations, more happiness for who you are and what you have. Choose gratitude for the gift of life! And at the end of the day, let's all be thankful that our gifts are bigger than our problems.

Now, let's learn how detoxification treatments can galvanize your youth and vitality.

References Chapter 6:

1. "Life Expectancy at Birth by Race and Sex, 1930-2010." Infoplease. © 2000-2017 Sandbox Networks, Inc., publishing as Infoplease. 1 Jul. 2018 <https://www.infoplease.com/life-expectancy-birth-race-and-sex-1930-2010/>.
2. Heard, E., and R. A. Martienssen, "Transgenerational Epigenetic Inheritance: Myths and Mechanisms," *Cell* (2014);157(1):95-109.
3. Singh S., and S. S. Li, "Epigenetic Effects of Environmental Chemicals Bisphenol A and Phthalates." *International Journal of Molecular Sciences* (2012);13(8): 10143–10153.
4. Waddington C. H., "The Epigenotype," *Endeavour* (1942a);1:18–20.
5. Willett, W. C., "Balancing Life-Style and Genomics Research for Disease Prevention," *Science* (2002);296(5568):695–698.

CHAPTER 7
YOUR DETOX FOR MENOPAUSE

The Body's Detoxification System

In today's highly polluted world, it has become imperative to have a diet and lifestyle that support your body's natural ability to detox. Oftentimes, our clients do not realize that the body has its own internal, hourly detoxification system working hard to keep them feeling well and looking great. Let's briefly examine three of the most critical organs involved in the body's detoxification system.

The Liver

How many times have you heard someone say (or said it to yourself), "My liver is going hate me!" after a night out drinking and making poor food choices? The truth is your liver does not get "emotionally" upset with you, but it does have to work overtime to remove all the toxins. It is not just the alcohol and junk foods that your liver is dealing with—hopefully only occasionally. But the liver has to process *everything* we consume (food, water, medications, the air we breathe) and put onto our bodies (beauty products) too. Its proper function even requires that we breathe correctly. You can imagine, it is a busy little liver.

The liver is the largest of our glands. It weighs between three to four pounds. It serves as the chemical factory in the body, and has over a hundred vital duties. For instance, it manufactures bile to aid in fat digestion. Bile then gets stored in the gallbladder and is released when we eat fatty foods. It also manufactures many of the enzymes that are critical in breaking down our food. The liver converts sugar into glycogen, a starch. It stores this excess glycogen until it is needed for energy by the body. It also breaks down hemoglobin, insulin, and other hormones. But of all of the hundreds of functions, the primary function of the liver—and most crucial to fat loss—is to act as a *filter*. It is a filter that cleans the blood of waste matter, mutated hormones, dead blood cells, fats, and chemical additives. It also filters out impurities or toxins that may result from the cooking or pasteurization of food. When the liver becomes strained and overworked, like any other part of our body, it slows down and starts to malfunction. A good example of alteration of one of its vital functions is its ability to break down and assimilate fat soluble vitamins (A, D, E, K, and F). If it's not functioning well, however, you may take vitamin supplements from now until your last breath, and the supplements will not work. Often clients come into our centers with bags of supplements they are taking (some take nearly fifty a day!). Once we have them complete a health history and symptom questionnaire, we find the problem is often with the liver and rarely what the symptoms alone would lead us to. Therefore, our program always has clients start with two weeks of a serious metabolic cleanse. This way we get your liver (and other detox organs: gut, kidneys, lungs, and skin) and the enzymes it produces working again so nutrients can move back into your cells. Our fourteen-day Metabolic Cleanse provides targeted nutrients that help your body gently dispose of the toxic buildup that has been accumulating for years. Cleansing acts as your first step toward improving liver function, improving your hormonal balance, and ultimately optimizing your fat loss goals.

After years of abuse and use, your liver, in particular, may grow sluggish. In middle age, between the ages of thirty-five to fifty-five, most women move less while eating and drinking as they did when they were younger and far more active. So the liver, which thrives on fresh organic foods and healthy amounts of movement, may not function optimally.

Common symptoms include headaches, fatigue, gas, bloating, acid reflux, and a general feeling of misery and malaise. Without regular exercise, limited chemical exposure, and enough fresh organic green vegetables and fruits, even a teetotaler can develop a suboptimal liver. You simply cannot persistently abuse the liver and maintain good health and be free from disease. Progressively, the whole body suffers, including your best attempts at weight loss.

The Colon

The next critical organ involved in detoxification is the colon. The colon is a section of your large intestines where solid waste residue is received through the process of digestion. A healthy functioning colon regularly eliminates solid waste, which cannot be used by the body nutritionally, as feces through the rectum. The colon contains both "good" (probiotics) and "bad" bacteria which are either working to maintain our health or working to destroy it. Good bacteria enhances health and is beneficial to the body. Bad bacteria can attack our body's cells or produce toxins that cause disease or infection (even death). We need both types of bacteria, but a much higher ratio (close to 85 percent) of the "good" to sustain optimal digestive health and immune function (Benno 1986, 13-25; Grönlund 2000, 186-192). You also need this balance to keep your bowels flowing regularly.

Trouble occurs when too much food or food that is too rich does not get fully digested by the "good" bacteria. The undigested food particles are turned into toxins that, through bacteria action, render the fats rancid. The carbohydrates start to ferment in the stomach (a common cause of acid reflux), and the protein putrefies (Choe et al. 2017, 363–369). When these toxic food particles become impacted in the colon, we have a condition known as intestinal toxemia. This impacted waste consistently oozes through the semi-permeable wall of the colon into your bloodstream where it represents a permanent source of body pollution, inflammation, weight gain, weight loss resistance, and ultimately, sickness.

The Kidneys

Typically the kidneys don't get much attention in the whole detoxing sphere, but they are probably just as important to address as the colon and liver. The kidneys play a major role in filtering waste and toxins to maintain our internal environment in as ideal condition as possible. They work like a fine-tuned clock to constantly filter your blood and eliminate toxins in the form of urine. If you are prone to urinary tract infections, kidney stones, or fluid retention, you'll definitely benefit from a kidney flush. You are in luck, as our program targets cleansing the kidneys in addition to the colon and liver. Our B3H+ Metabolic Cleanse protocol combines a customized nutritional kidney cleanse diet (high in electrolytes and antioxidants to help heal the kidneys) with specific herbal supplements. What's really incredible is, if you follow our protocol, you'll feel your energy levels skyrocket as a result of improved kidney function.

In summary, for your body's natural detoxification to work well on its own, you have to maintain the health and function of these three organs. You can keep these systems running smoothly by nourishing your body with "detoxifying" foods and supplemental support as needed.

Detoxing to Lose

To effectively lose weight and keep it off, you should be regularly flushing your body of toxins. The more toxic you become, the less effective your body will be at absorbing and processing nutrients and fats. The latest research suggests that chronic chemical exposure and waste products wreak havoc on our health by making us fat and more likely to become diabetic (Zeliger 2013, 9–20).

How do these toxic substances make us fat when they contain no calories? It's simple. Once toxins get into your body, these chemicals can disrupt your endocrine system. Your endocrine system consists of a network of glands (adrenal, ovaries, pancreas, thyroid, and so forth) that secrete chemical messengers (aka hormones) and other products, like enzymes, directly into the blood. When your endocrine system is overexposed to toxic trash, the chemical messages become altered or blocked. This de-regulation contributes to weight gain in a variety of ways. It slows the metabolism; interferes with thyroid hormone signaling; inhibits your ability to absorb nutrients, break down cholesterol, stabilize blood sugars; and increases risk for leptin and insulin resistance (diabetes) (Soto 2010, 363–370; Patrick 2009, 326–346; Tuma 2007, 835).

Another way toxic overload makes people fat—and sick—is by expanding the size or number of adipose cells (fat cells) and stuffing them full of toxic trash along with the fat. This is the body's way of keeping these harmful foreign chemicals away from key organs. This causes easy fat gain and makes losing weight that much more difficult because your body does not want to release toxic fat into circulation where it could accelerate the onset of aging and disease (Tuma 2007, 835).

A key to a healthy metabolism, immune, and hormonal system is through the endocrine system. You see, the endocrine system, together with the nervous system (and primary detox organs) are designed to keep us healthy and vigorous with age. If our diets, lifestyle, and environment are not free of stress and poisonous chemicals, the glands will suffer and provoke weight gain and other symptoms and diseases. Although, if the endocrine glands are functioning properly, you need never grow old, sick, or fat.

Breathe Deep to Detox

The easiest, quickest, and most cost-effective way to detox is through your breath. Deep diaphragmatic breathing has been shown to gently massage the liver (and other internal organs, such as the stomach, small intestines, and pancreas) as a natural consequence of its action (Li 2002, 50; Limongi et al. 2016, 429–436). Yet, seldom do we consider breathing to positively affect our liver function.

Shallow breathing fails to give the liver this continuous massage effect it needs to keep fit. Thus, our vital life support system (our breath) becomes a factor in a malfunctioning liver. Breathing correctly oxidizes the blood and invigorates our organs (Limongi et al. 2016, 429–436).

Practice slow, deep-breathing in and out through the nose for at least five to ten minutes a day to assist in detoxifying your liver and body. There's a bonus—this practice can also relieve perceived stress and helps lower anxiety by calming your nervous system and slowing down your heart rate.

Knowing When It's Time to Detox

Here I present a list of some of the major signs of toxic overload and how the symptoms may present themselves in the body. If you have more than three that *persistently* cause problematic symptoms, and you are over the age forty, it's probably an ideal time to detox.

- Excessive weight or obesity
- Hormonal irregularities
- Skin conditions (for example, acne)
- Food allergies or sensitivities
- Congestion or chronic excess mucus
- Bloating or abnormal fluid retention
- Intestinal issues
- Arthritis (or aches in joints)
- Cognitive issues (forgetfulness, lack of focus)
- Mood swings
- Chronic infections
- Sleep disorders
- Stress (unmanaged)
- Rapid aging
- Severe PMS or menopausal symptoms
- High blood pressure
- Diabetes
- Low energy
- General lethargy or malaise (for example, "I just don't feel well")

Health and Beauty Benefits of Detoxification

The beneficial effects of detoxification are directly conveyed to every organ, gland, cell, muscle, and joint in the body. When done regularly, it helps us avoid the toxic overload before it becomes a major health problem. Cleanse your body of toxic trash and prevent the necessary buildup of additional noxious elements through a planned, individually tailored protocol devised by our medical and nutrition experts. In planning, they can take into account your particular lifestyle, nutritional habits, personal preferences, and general physical health. You'll see immediately that this type of treatment significantly differs from so-called "crash" detoxification that is not conducive to your long-term health.

The major benefits of the B3H+ Metabolic Cleanse are as follows:

- Helps you lose weight faster than without detoxing
- Assists in balancing hormones
- Cleanses the liver, colon, kidneys
- Eliminates free radicals, chemical pollutants, and toxins caused by bacteria (for example, acute and chronic viral infections) by boosting the immune system
- Boosts energy
- Supports digestion
- Reduces stress
- Improves concentration
- Improves mood
- Increases circulation, which promotes healthier, glowing skin
- Helps lower systemic inflammation
- Aids in removal of heavy metals, especially lead and mercury toxicity, which is caused by ingesting farmed fish and by amalgams (tooth fillings)

Finally, toxins are ubiquitous in today's society. There is no escaping their reach. In addition, it may seem like an unattainable goal to avoid them all. We understand. But if you want to lose weight and regain hormonal harmony, your youthful look, and your energy, you need to take simple measures to counteract your exposure to harmful chemicals. So, we made this easy by highlighting our favorite tips to optimize your body's natural detoxification process.

1. **Eat foods rich in vitamin C.** Fruits and vegetables rich in vitamin C help reduce the damage caused by heavy metal toxins by acting as antioxidants. The fruits and vegetables highest in vitamin C include: bananas, cantaloupe, raw kale, and broccoli.

2. **Eat garlic and onions.** Keep the vampires away and your liver healthy by eating these two potent sulfur-rich detoxifiers. Other foods that aid in detoxification and are excellent sources of sulfur include the cruciferous vegetables—broccoli, kale, brussel sprouts, collard greens, and cabbage.

3. **Drink lemon water.** Drinking clean, high-quality spring water with lemon throughout the day (especially first thing in the morning) helps flush out toxins that are released while you are going through your cleansing phase. Lemon water is also alkalizing to the body. Drink it hot or tepid. And try it with fresh ginger.

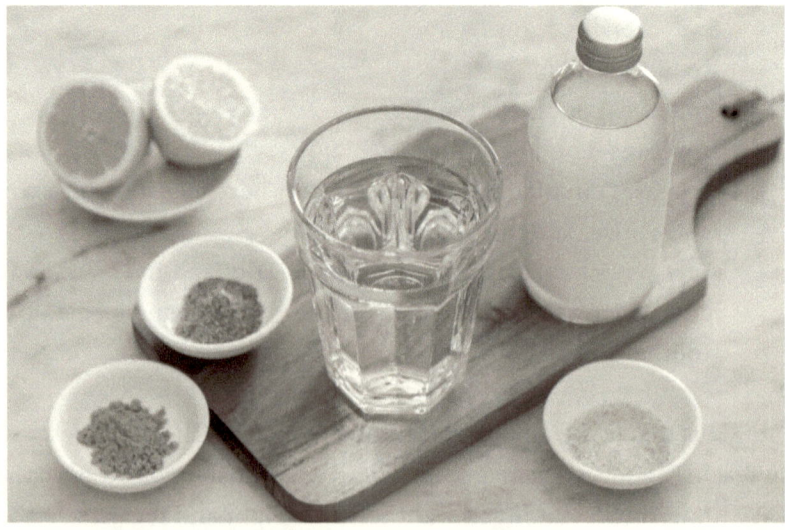

4. **Twist it out.** Twisting poses (at the trunk of the body), like the ones you'd do in yoga, aid liver detoxification and stimulate digestion.

5. **Go organic.** If it's financially feasible, eat primarily organic foods, since many pesticides are indeed endocrine (or hormone) disruptors (see the "dirty dozen" list in chapter 4).

6. **Love your liver.** Avoid foods or drinks that are highly refined or processed; break a sweat daily through various modes of exercise; breathe deeply; talk with a holistic health professional for recommendations on vitamins, minerals, and enzyme liver support.

7. **Keep your cells healthy.** We all have both antioxidants and free radicals circulating in our bodies at all times. Some antioxidants are synthesized by our bodies. Some we get by eating a diet high in antioxidant foods, which double as anti-inflammatory foods. Others we must get by taking supplements. Free radicals are natural byproducts of cellular reactions. But, if the body is placed under prolonged stress from things like poor nutrition, some medications, or exposure to toxins, certain types of oxygen molecules travel freely in the body which may cause oxidative damage to cells (Uttara et al. 2009, 65–74). This oxidative stress manufactures excess free radicals which accelerate aging, damage tissue, mutate cells (causing certain cancers), and negatively alter genes (DNA) and our immune system. More than ever, and because we are all aging and exposed to some amount of oxidative damage, we need to supplement with antioxidants, whole-food nutrients, and phytonutrients to boost our immune systems. This is why we created a specific supplement line that provides a concentrated source of antioxidants and rich phytonutrients. This daily immune boost reduces oxidative stress, fights free radical damage, and protects healthy cells while halting the growth of malignant and cancerous cells.

8. **Ditch plastics.** Avoid eating and drinking out of BPA plastic-lined cans or containers. Buy microwave-safe glass or stoneware to heat food,

and use glass or stainless steel water bottles to carry around with you. We love the insulated, stainless steel water bottles made by Hydro Flask in Bend, Oregon (www.hydroflask.com). Also, limit the handling of your cash register receipts, which now are coated in BPA. Ask for an electronic receipt or have your paper receipt placed into the bag instead of into your hand.

9. **Use only natural makeup and cleaning products.** This is where you'll find some of the biggest culprits of endocrine-disrupting chemicals. A good rule of thumb when it comes to beauty products is: If you can't eat it, you should avoid putting it on your body.

Final Words

We cannot stress often enough that your body will not handle systemic overload. Eventually, your immune system will fail and ill health and added pounds will bog you down. But this does not have to be anyone's fate. To maintain a high state of health and a beautiful, younger, stronger, leaner body resistant to disease, it is essential to consume living, organic foods rather than foods treated with added chemicals and preservatives. In addition, it's critical to lower your exposure to world pollutants by using natural, chemical-free products in your home and on your body. Finally, the best drinking waters for detoxifying are clean, safe, high-quality spring waters or alkalizing mineral water.

Are you ready now to give The B3H+ Metabolic Cleanse a try? We know you'll find it is an effective detoxification protocol that will improve the internal and external environment and health of your body. Plus, it kick-starts weight loss before you begin Phase 2's Lean Body Plan. When they follow our instructions, most clients lose five pounds safely and relatively easily during the fourteen-day detox. They also experience increased energy, reduced cravings, and an overall improvement in their well-being.

References Chapter 7:

1. Benno, Y., and T. Mitsuoka, "Development of Intestinal Microflora in Humans and Animals," *Bifidobateria Microflora* (1986);5:13–25.
2. Choe, J. W., et al., "Foods Inducing Typical Gastroesophageal Reflux Disease Symptoms in Korea," *Journal of Neurogastroenterology and Motility* (2017);23: 363-369.
3. Grönlund, M. M., et al., "Importance of Intestinal Colonisation in The Maduration of Humoral Immunity in Early Infancy: A Prospective Follow Up Study of Healthy Infants Aged 0-6 Months," *Archives of Disease in Childhood* (2000);83:186–192.
4. Li, M., K. Chen, and Z. Mo, "Use of Qigong Therapy in the Detoxification of Heroin Addicts," *Alternative Therapies in Health and Medicine* (2002);8(1):50.
5. Limongi, V., et al., "Exercise Manual for Liver Disease Patients," *World Journal of Transplantation* 6.2 (2016):429–436.
6. Patrick L., "Thyroid Disruption: Mechanism and Clinical Implications in Human Health," *Alternative Medicine Review* (2009);14(4):326-46.
7. Soto, A. M., and C. Sonnenschein, "Environmental Causes of Cancer: Endocrine Disruptors as Carcinogens," *Nature Reviews Endocrinology* (2010); 6(7):363-370.
8. Tuma, S., "Environmental Chemicals—Not Just Overeating—May Cause Obesity," *Journal of the National Cancer Institute* (2007);99(11):835.
9. Uttara, Bayani, et al. "Oxidative Stress and Neurodegenerative Diseases: A Review of Upstream and Downstream Antioxidant Therapeutic Options," *Current Neuropharmacology* 7.1 (2009):65–74.
10. Zeliger, H., "Lipophilic Chemical Exposure as a Cause of Type 2 Diabetes (T2D)," *Reviews on Environmental Health* (2013);28(1):9–20.

CHAPTER 8
REBALANCING A LOW-FUNCTIONING THYROID

A Road to Recovery

The thyroid gland's systematic function in midlife health is regulation of body weight, hormonal balance, and disease. This function is frequently misunderstood. The topic of thyroid health is particularly baffling and concerning to our female clients as they have a substantially higher susceptibility than men to develop a thyroid disorder. In fact, middle-aged women are five to eight times more likely than men to experience thyroid problems, especially after a big hormonal event like menopause (Shinkov et al. 2014, 269). Poor performance of the thyroid interferes with body temperature, which slows metabolism, often reducing the ability to maintain a comfortable weight and energy.

ad any of the form

	Diabetes
	High cholesterol
✓	Thyroid problem
	Hepatitis

members of family affected)
| | Diabetes |

If you have a thyroid disorder that has made you gain additional weight, you may have encountered ridicule, humiliation, or harsh judgment from others. We've had clients share that people say things like "You are just lazy" or "You need to eat less, exercise more" or "Try harder." Yet, they have tried everything to stop the weight gain. Some have been willing to pay almost any price, have tried every diet imaginable, and exercised religiously despite low energy trying to prevent more weight gain. Can you relate? If you say yes, please don't lose hope of ever losing the weight. What you probably need is some help identifying and correcting a low-functioning thyroid and following our hormone reset, not another diet.

It's particularly disturbing to hear that women's doctors often tell them they are not trying hard enough. No matter what changes they make, they feel tired and cold all the time and can't keep their weight at an appropriate level for their body size. To us, it sounds like a thyroid disorder, yet their annual blood panel suggests their thyroid has tested normal again. Thus, their doctor does not recognize their low thyroid function, and it goes untreated for a longer period of time.

Most of our largest clients are not overeating, consuming junk pseudo-foods, or under exercising. If anything, many of them are under eating because eating in moderation and exercising have resulted in excess weight gain. In an effort to understand what's going on, we decided to look at the research on long-term success rates on the country's most popular diet programs. We discovered that the majority of women who are not losing fat by cutting calories are not overeating. We also found the dropout rates for these popular programs is around 65 to 75 percent at 12 weeks, partly because dieters cannot lose fat by cutting calories alone (Neve 2010, 69).

As you learned in chapter 2, the traditional calorie-in, calorie-out approach rarely produces sustainable weight loss. Years of calorie restriction and yo-yo dieting may have also triggered adaptive thermogenesis, in which the metabolic rate decreases to compensate for the lower caloric intake. Thus, when you quit restricting calories, and return to your "normal" eating habits from before you lost the weight, you quickly store more calories as fat because of a lower metabolic set point (Leibel et al. 1995, 621–628). What you'll discover in this chapter is that low-calorie dieting also suppresses thyroid function, causing more calories to be stored as fat instead of burned as fuel. For most women, dieting just makes their sluggish thyroid more sluggish. When this happens, it can't take cues from other hormones (like leptin, nature's appetite suppressant) to maintain a body weight set point. So many people with a sluggish thyroid also suffer from a deficit in leptin signaling because their bodies are leptin resistant (Zimmermann-Belsing et al. 2003, 257–271). In terms of weight loss, leptin works directly with the thyroid to stimulate the release of critical hormones which break down fat (Zimmermann-Belsing et al. 2003, 257–271).

Our medical director, Dr. Siobhan Kealy, and her staff can help you identify why your thyroid isn't functioning properly. You'll be able to make real changes that make a difference in your health, hormones, and weight. To further help you understand why your thyroid is functioning subpar in midlife, let's look at it a bit closer.

Thyroid 101

Where is your thyroid? The thyroid gland is the largest of your endocrine glands. It's shaped like a butterfly and sits at the base of your neck on your vocal cords.

What does the thyroid do? The thyroid is a remarkable master gland that has operation over virtually every cell and system in your body. Its most critical function is regulating cell metabolism like a thermostat. Your cells will function completely differently if you are burning hot or freezing cold. When your thyroid function is low (what is called hypothyroidism), it will not produce enough active hormones; neither will its cells hear signals from other hormones (like, thyroid stimulating hormone [TSH] or leptin). Or your immune system may be attacking your thyroid's own tissues (the most common thyroid condition is Hashimoto's thyroiditis). As a result, your whole system becomes under active or inactive. Which is exactly the way you will feel. Literally, every part of your body—your hair, skin, heart, joints, brain and on and on—is diminished when the thyroid is not performing well. And metabolism is affected as well.

Symptoms of Low Thyroid Function (Hypothyroidism)

First and foremost, if you suspect you have a thyroid problem, carefully look yourself at your symptoms and blood work results as well as your family and personal health histories. We find that, even if a test result comes back normal, your sense of something not functioning properly in your body is a good indicator that something is wrong.

When you start the B3H+ metabolic weight-loss program, our doctors do a physical examination of your thyroid, request and review a body temperature log, and order a comprehensive female hormone panel in which more than a dozen markers are tested and reviewed. Our complete hormone panel includes a full metabolic panel with lipids, cortisol, leptin, TSH, free T4 and free T3 (active thyroid hormone, which is converted from free T4), reverse T3 (a metabolic hormone that, when produced in excess, blocks your thyroid receptors and prevents free T3 from getting into your cells), and thyroid antibodies, plus thyroid blockers (such as toxins and heavy metals), DHEA-S (a steroid hormone produced by the adrenal hormone, often getting very low in cases of hypothyroidism), as well as the two building blocks of thyroid hormones (tyrosine and iodine). Additionally, we do a complete check of your sex hormones: estrogen, estradiol, pregnenolone, progesterone, and total and free testosterone.

We advise that clients begin testing their thyroid markers annually starting around age forty or sooner if they have several of the most common symptoms or have any that are severe. Having this history of what thyroid function looks like can be very informative and helpful in case of thyroid changes. At minimum, ask your doctor to run the full panel of thyroid tests, not just TSH and T4 the inactive form. Also, make sure you are tested for free T3, reverse T3, and thyroid antibodies (TPO and Tg) so you get the clearest picture of what inflammation may be going on inside the body. If your doctor refuses to do a comprehensive panel, you'll want to find either another doctor or a functional medicine practitioner who can test and asses your results and symptoms.

The complete thyroid panel should include:

- TSH
- Free T4
- Free T3 (Most Important)
- Reverse T3 and the two Hashimoto's antibodies
- TPO (thyroid peroxidase)
- TG (thyroglobulin)

Along with these six, you will want your vitamin D-25 hydroxy, B12, B6, ferritin (iron storage), and DHEA tested.

To find a list of your local medical professionals specializing in thyroid function and the latest treatments through diet, medicine, and lifestyle check out:

- Paleo Physicians Network: www.paleophysiciansnetwork.com
- Naturopathic Medicine Network: www.pandamedicine.com

We encourage self-investigation and gathering a copious amount information about your thyroid and diagnosis and then interpreting your test results and considering controllable lifestyle factors. Self-knowledge is empowering, and taking action is key to understanding the effects of your condition on your health and how it can be treated and corrected using an integrative approach. There are a several books we suggest:

- *The Thyroid Connection: Why You Feel Tired, Brain-Fogged, and Overweight—and How to Get Your Life Back* by Amy Myers, M.D.
- *Stop the Thyroid Madness II: How Thyroid Experts Are Challenging Ineffective treatments and Improving the Lives of Patients* by over are a dozen insightful medical doctors
- *Why do I still have Thyroid Symptoms? When My Lab Test are Normal: A Revolutionary Breakthrough in Understanding Hashimoto's Disease* by Dr. Datis Kharrazian, DHSc, D.C., MS

- *Thyroid and Menopausal Madness: Why It Feels Like You're Falling Apart and What You Can Do About It* by Joni Labbe, D.C.
- *Recovering with T3: My Journey from Hypothyroidism to Good Health Using the T3 Thyroid Hormone* (forward by Dr. John C. Lowe) by Paul Robinson

The most common symptoms of low thyroid function include:

- Slow metabolism—unexplainable weight gain or inability to lose weight
- Cold hands and feet due to decrease in body temperature (below 97.8 degrees)
- Low energy, fatigue, not feeling rested after many hours of sleep
- Dry or scaly skin
- Joint or muscular pain
- Hair loss
- Dry, coarse hair
- Voice changes, particularly raspy or hoarse sounding
- Constipation and feeling bloated
- Foggy brain
- Depression and moodiness
- Menstrual problems, including heavier periods, irregular period and severe PMS
- Goiters (very rare)

Multiple Reasons for Low Thyroid Function

Under normal conditions, the hypothalamus in the brain produces thyroid-stimulating hormone (TSH) in the pituitary gland. TSH stimulates the thyroid to produce thyroxine (total T4), which is then converted to its sister hormone triiodothyronine (total T3). Total T3, which are thyroid hormones bound to proteins, is then converted into free T3 (active, usable form) hormones unbound from the proteins, which allows them to actually enter the cells and do their job. If free T3 can't get into cells, thyroid symptoms appear. Since free T3 has the greatest effect on the body's metabolism, intestinal function, temperature, brain function, and other hormones, it actually must be present on every cell in the body to activate our genes, which influences how well we work on the inside.

Hypothyroidism signals an underactive thyroid, a dysfunction that derives from a deficiency in the production of the thyroid hormone and may either be caused by primary or secondary reasons. Primary hypothyroidism occurs when the thyroid does not make sufficient amounts of thyroid hormones. It is usually characterized by a high normal or high TSH and low free T4 and low T3.

The most common cause of primary hypothyroidism is an autoimmune disease called Hashimoto's thyroiditis. In fact, Hashimoto's is the most common form of autoimmune disease in the United States, affecting more than 10 percent of women over thirty, and women are ten times more likely to develop the condition than men (Skugor 2009, 11–28; Canaris et al. 2000, 526–534). With Hashimoto's, the immune system attacks the thyroid gland as if it were a foreign tissue or invader in the body.

According to the Mayo Clinic website (http://www.mayoclinic.com), studies suggest that about 90 percent of people with hypothyroidism are producing antibodies that are mistakenly trying to destroy the thyroid gland and its hormones. It is also possible to develop primary hypothyroidism from non-autoimmune reasons. The Mayo Clinic website lists other possible causes: iodine deficiency, obesity, mutations in TSH receptors, non-thyroid chronic diseases, damage to the thyroid, or removal of the thyroid (at times due to cancer).

On the other hand, secondary hypothyroidism is caused by a disorder in the pituitary gland or hypothalamus in the brain. It is much less common than the primary forms, and is usually characterized by low or low-normal TSH, and low free T4 and T3.

Whether your thyroid is under attack from your own immune system or you have the non-autoimmune form of low thyroid dysfunction, you'll want to change your diet and add nutritional supplements to help. Many of you will need to consult a functional medicine doctor who specializes in thyroid and other endocrine problems. This is the ideal type of specialist to test your thyroid hormones, thyroid antibodies (in case of Hashimoto's), and decipher what is causing your thyroid disorder. They'll know what supplements may help and if you need further support from thyroid medicine.

How Entering Menopause Could Trigger Low Thyroid Function

During perimenopause and menopause, the whole body goes through serious hormonal changes. This hormonal event is enough to throw many vulnerable women into low thyroid states. Low thyroid, which slows metabolism, often leads to unwanted weight gain.

There is also a close interrelationship between thyroid and sex hormone function. The slowing of metabolism slows reproductive organ function as well. One of the main changes occurs in the ovaries where there is a decreased production of sex hormones, progesterone, estrogen, and testosterone. The major drops and imbalances in sex hormones dramatically impacts how the body's cells respond to thyroid hormones. For instance, progesterone has multiple functions in thyroid health. They include the promotion of the assimilation of thyroid hormones into the cells, which gives you abundant energy. Research also suggests progesterone helps synthesize (and increases) free T4 which is required to make sufficient amounts of free T3 (active, usable form).

When you transition into perimenopause, progesterone levels begin to fall in advance of estrogen, causing a state of estrogen dominance. If left unbalanced for too long, undesirable side effects can appear (revisit chapter 2 to review high estrogen symptoms). This imbalance of low progesterone relative to high estrogen causes the liver to produce high levels of a protein called "thyroid-binding globulin," which, as its name suggests, binds the thyroid hormone and reduces the amount of thyroid hormone (free T3) that can be assimilated into and used by the cells. This is one of the biggest triggers for low thyroid function for women entering middle age.

Another potential hormonal trigger, specifically linked to Hashimoto's autoimmune disease, are the erratic swings in estrogen before women transition into menopause. These fluctuations can turn on the gene expression for Hashimoto's in the presence of inflammation, genetic susceptibility, and gut permeability. In addition, increases in estrogen have been shown to exacerbate the immune system's attack on the thyroid (Amino et al. 2003, 815–818). This may explain the rise of early thyroid autoimmune conditions during perimenopause, a time when estrogen is wildly fluctuating.

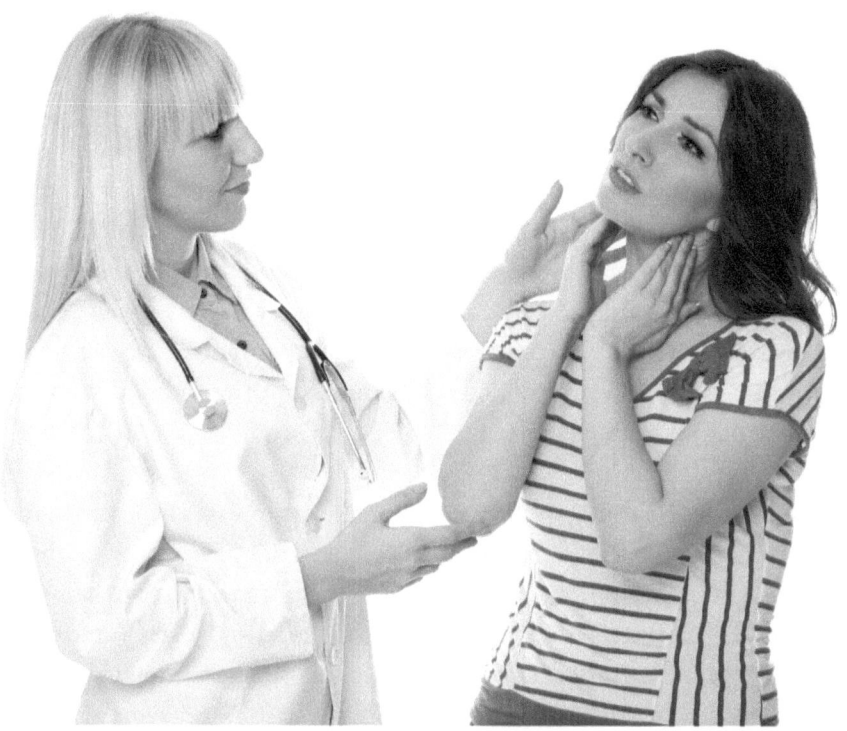

Many of the symptoms of low thyroid and menopausal changes are interrelated. A simple complaint to your doctor that you are anxious, gaining weight, tired, cold, or depressed will likely lead to treatments or remedies that address the symptoms only. For instance, antidepressant medications are often prescribed to help balance mood. Unfortunately, this protocol ignores or misdiagnoses the problem of a dysfunctional thyroid. In addition, doctors who still practice outdated, conventional thyroid diagnoses and treatments perform only a single lab test, which typically includes TSH and maybe T4. If you fall into the "normal" ranges, chances are your problem will be overlooked or misdiagnosed again. In order to uncover the causes of your thyroid troubles, it is imperative to get a complete thyroid panel and antibody test.

Other Common Triggers of Low Thyroid Function

1. **Soy**—When it comes to your thyroid, there is no joy in eating soy. Today, soy is one of the most genetically modified crops in America, and it is sprayed with dozens of poisonous chemicals to keep it growing strong. Today's soy is no health food; it's complete garbage. When consumed daily, it increases TSH and can depress thyroid function by disrupting the conversion of T4 to free T3 (Silverstein et al. 2014, 1136–1142). Sadly, most soy can trigger an autoimmune response in the body, leading to an attack on the thyroid tissue and hormones. Also, because soy is a phytoestrogen (plant source of estrogen, which mimics estrogen in the body), it can disrupt thyroid and hormone balance for both genders.

2. **Low-calorie diets**—Chronic dieting also depresses healthy thyroid function. How? When you frequently restrict calories (which your body senses as starvation), the thyroid slows metabolism to help hold onto its nutritional resources until the "food shortage" (dieting) is over. Many chronic dieters suffer from this compensation (lowering) in their metabolism until their thyroid condition is corrected through a restorative diet, thyroid supplements, medication, and typically, hormone replacement therapy. They also suffer from the results of permanently slowing down their metabolic fire by gaining post diet unwanted pounds.

3. **Chronic gut inflammation**—The gut is your gateway to optimal or poor health. Gut inflammation is caused primarily by certain irritating foods, which leads to gut permeability, also called "leaky gut."

What does leaky gut mean? In simple terms, it means that the barrier (or wall) between your small intestines and blood stream is compromised and substances that should stay inside the intestines are now directly passing into the bloodstream. Here is an analogy: Imagine the walls of small intestines as a brick barrier with mortar between each brick. When you consume, let's say, your pastry for breakfast, which contains wheat gluten (and refined sugar and probably some other pseudo food substances), the mortar between each brick gets chipped away a little bit at a time. Each time you eat gluten-containing foods, the mortar breaks away again and again, until these tight "mortar-like" junctions between the bricks become gaping holes, creating intestinal permeability (aka leaky gut). This can also be caused or exacerbated by too much stress, dairy products, antibiotics, NSAIDs, toxins, and some medications like birth control.

Now that the gut wall is compromised, toxins, microbes, undigested proteins, and food particles can pass directly into the bloodstream. This sets off an alarm signaling your immune system that foreign invaders need to be destroyed. Immediately your immune system goes into action to neutralize the situation, creating inflammatory chemicals and antibodies to attack. Unfortunately, over time this inflammatory response to the threat from outside invaders puts you on a pathway to autoimmune diseases. These develop because your immune system is stressed and overworked. At this point, it gets confused and mistakenly attacks your thyroid tissues, which have a similar molecular structure to the structure of the foreign invaders. This causes an autoimmune thyroid disease such as Hashimoto's thyroiditis or Graves' disease.

The main culprits of leaky gut are wheat and other gluten-containing grains specifically known to cause and exacerbate the symptoms of Hashimoto's, dairy (especially casein proteins), phytates, and lectins (in certain gluten-free grains and beans). If you have leaky gut, these foods can set off a chain reaction that leads to both autoimmune hypothyroidism and non-autoimmune thyroid disease. At minimum, if you have any autoimmune disease or think you may, avoid gluten and cow dairy, the most problematic foods (Vojdani 2013, 20–32).

4. **Carbohydrates too low**— We agree with the consensus to eliminate all gluten-containing grains and limiting sugar, junk foods, and other poor-quality sources of carbohydrates, but women must be cautious with carb restriction. Excessively low carb (less than 50 grams per day) or no-carb diets have been shown to lead to thyroid problems, adrenal issues, mood swings, cravings, hunger, and energy dips. The main reason that carbohydrates affect thyroid function directly is that insulin is needed for the conversion of inactive T4 to active T3, and insulin is typically kept low on a low-carbohydrate diet. For these reasons, we encourage our clients with thyroid and adrenal issues to moderately consume low-sugar fruit, gluten-free grains (if tolerable), sweet potatoes, squash, and beans (see the carbohydrate threshold chart in this chapter).

5. **Poor Adrenal Function (too much stress!)**— Many women with thyroid problems also have exhausted adrenal function. If you tend to feel "tired but wired" or become more alert in the evenings but exhausted in the mornings, become overwhelmed easily, experience strong cravings or feelings of hunger shortly after you've eaten a meal, your adrenals may also be contributing to your problems. The adrenals and the thyroid work closely together. If the thyroid function fails, the adrenals have to work harder to keep you energized. Eventually, they'll run out of steam too. It works in the opposite direction too. If the adrenals are working overtime to deal with high levels of stress (perceived or real), your thyroid turns everything down to keep your system calm. Thus, you can clearly see there is a delicate balance between your thyroid function and your adrenal glands.

    It's time for all of us to seriously manage our stress better with meditation or yoga, more time for hobbies and other enjoyable activities, a good night's rest, massage, hot baths, infrared sauna, walks in nature, or whatever brings you the most peace and joy. In addition, many need to begin reducing their dependence on caffeinated products, which increases the release of stress hormones.

6. **Genetics**— Your genes influence your susceptibility for an autoimmune thyroid disease like Hashimoto's disease or Grave's disease, which are caused by the hyperfunction of the thyroid gland. However, none of the immune regulatory genes associated with the disease necessarily equates to a development of an autoimmune thyroid disease. It appears that development is linked more to the powerful interaction of your genes and your environment (food, lifestyle, habits, toxic load, and so forth) (Davies et al. 2012, 6). If you have family members who have been diagnosed or are being treated for hypothyroidism (and even non-autoimmune hypothyroidism), we suggest you review your symptoms with them in mind and interview them if they are open to discussion. You may be surprised at what you can learn from their experiences. Also, it would be wise to share the genetic and family history with your doctor.

7. **Iodine deficiency**—Thyroid hormones are made up from the amino-acid tyrosine and iodine. Tyrosine is easily found through most forms of animal protein. Iodine was (and is) a bit harder to find. In the early 1940s iodine deficiency was thought to be the biggest contributor to the rapid increase in thyroid disorders (notably, disfiguring goiters in the neck) due to depleted soils in the United States. In response, iodized salt was added to our food system to remedy this epidemic. Unfortunately, we learned that all this iodized salt contributed to an increased risk for autoimmune hypothyroidism, which has continued to plague us worldwide and aggravate autoimmune symptoms. Today iodine deficiency is much less common in the industrialized world and much less a cause of hypothyroidism. But the research in this area is inconclusive and is still in progress. It is ideal to get your levels checked by a doctor who specializes in thyroid problems to determine if your specific situation requires iodine support. The healthiest foods rich in iodine are the edible sea vegetables. There are many varieties

including seaweeds like red, brown, and green algae; kelp; dulse; and nori. Try incorporating them into dishes such as soups, salads, beans, and even healthy desserts.

Maximizing Your Thyroid's Health

Up until now you've learned to identify your own sluggish thyroid symptoms and which of the two most common types of thyroid problems you may have—non-autoimmune hypothyroidism and Hashimoto's thyroiditis. You have also learned the importance of finding a helpful (holistic functional) thyroid doctor who can order the full panel of tests you need to confirm a diagnosis and customize your treatment. Now you are ready to discover how you can maximize your thyroid's health through thyroid-targeted nutrients and supplements.

Nutritional Support

In order to repair the symptoms of low thyroid function, an immediate change in diet is required. Another short-lived diet will not do the trick. Our nutritionists at B3H+ will help you make healthy nutrition a way of life, so that you can either prevent or assist in healing your thyroid condition and metabolism. If you have thyroid disease symptoms, you will need high quality foods and some basic nutritional supplements. To treat a sluggish thyroid and Hashimoto's, be sure you consume micronutrients, clean proteins, foods rich in Vitamin D, high-fiber vegetables, and fermentable fiber foods daily and eliminate gluten, soy, and dairy.

Micronutrients

Eat foods rich in micronutrients such as selenium, magnesium, B6, iron, and zinc (and possibly iodine, but note that iodine is not usually recommended if you have Hashimoto's). A deficiency in any of these elements has been linked to a variety of autoimmune disorders. The chronic inflammation associated with autoimmune conditions depletes the body of these vital nutrients This causes a cascade of problems as they are needed for optimizing the production and conversion of thyroid hormones.

Top food sources of micronutrients: Just two brazil nuts a day provides a good source of all these nutrients, especially selenium. Also include oysters, pumpkins seed, pistachios and other varieties of raw nuts and seeds into your diet daily.

Clean Proteins

Most protein sources provide high amounts of iron and vitamins A and K. These strengthen the immune system and help to balance hormones. Aim to consume at least one gram of protein per kilogram of body weight. To find your weight in kilograms, divide your weight in pounds by 2.2; for example, if you weigh 160 pounds, you should aim to eat around 72 grams of protein per day (around 20 to 25 grams per meal, which is equivalent to 3 to 4 ounces of fish, beef, fowl, or a vegan or vegetarian source).

Top food sources of vitamin A: True vitamin A is found only in animal products … like shellfish, fish, fermented cod liver oil, grass-fed beef, butter or ghee from grass-fed cows, and organ meats. The conversion rate from plant sources of vitamin A is very low, but that doesn't mean you should dismiss the idea of obtaining vitamin A through veggies with the highest contents, which include kale, collard greens, and broccoli.

Top food sources of vitamin K: Butter or ghee and organ meats from grass-fed beef are top sources of vitamin K. The best vegetarian sources of K are kale, collard greens, and natto, a Japanese superfood made from fermented soybeans (make sure it is non-GMO).

Top foods sources of iron: Grass-fed beef, especially liver. A vegetable source is spinach.

Optimize Vitamin D Levels

For decades, research has suggested a strong link between low levels of vitamin D and thyroid disorders. For example, we now know that people with low vitamin D levels have a higher risk for thyroid antibodies, which are found in both Grave's disease and Hashimoto's thyroiditis (Mackawy 2013, 267–275). In order to boost your immune system and thyroid function, which unlocks your fat-burning metabolism, increase your vitamin D level by sensible sun exposure (around fifteen minutes per day, or twenty to thirty minutes in the winter months, especially when living in areas of the country with fewer hours of light). If this is not enough or is not an option for you, then add a vitamin D3 supplement. If you supplement with vitamin D3, we recommend you take 2000 to 4000 IU per day with foods that are rich in healthy fats, such as avocado, nuts, extra virgin olive oil, or coconut oil. Also, it is critically important to heal a leaky gut in order to absorb the vitamin D you eat or supplement with.

Top food sources of vitamin D: Organic, free-range egg yolks, grass-fed beef liver, cod liver oil, and fatty fish such as salmon, sardines, herring, and mackerel.

High-Fiber Vegetables

Eat a wide variety of fruits and vegetables each day. The actual amount will depend on your body size. For example, a petite woman may eat four to five cups, and a two-hundred-pound man may eat nine cups or more. It's important to include nonstarchy, high-fiber green vegetables and colorful berries. Cruciferous veggies, in particular, are helpful for liver detoxification, balancing estrogen, improving immune function, reducing risk of several cancers, and reducing inflammation in the body. But clients often ask if eating cruciferous veggies will cause more thyroid problems. According to the research, if you are eating large amounts of sulfur-rich, cruciferous veggies and have an iodine deficiency (or hypothyroidism already) thyroid function may be inhibited (Truong et al. 2010, 1183–1192). So our advice, if you have a thyroid issue, is to consume cruciferous vegetables that have been cooked and limit your servings of these to one to two servings per day.

The most common cruciferous vegetables include: cabbage, spinach, broccoli, cauliflower, bok choy, arugula, turnip, kale, mustard and collard greens, brussel sprouts, watercress, and rutabaga.

Fermentable Fiber Foods

If you are eating four cups or more of veggies (preferred) and high-fiber fruits per day, you may be getting a sufficient amount of fermentable fiber in your diet. A fermentable fiber acts as a food source for your "good" gut bacteria, which in turn transforms it into short-chain fatty acids. These fatty acids enter the bloodstream and positively influence your immune system.

Top food sources of fermentable fibers: Chicory root, dandelion greens, garlic, onions, leeks, bananas, plantains, yams, sweet potatoes, and Jerusalem artichokes.

Gluten, Soy, and Dairy

Remove gluten for good. Wheat, rye, oats, and barley all contain gut-irritating gluten which is known to trigger an autoimmune thyroid disease (Roy et al. 2016, 880–890). If you have an autoimmune disease you will want to be 100 percent gluten free to prevent the immune destruction to your thyroid. Sorry folks, the 80/20 rule (80 percent of the time you don't eat gluten-containing foods but 20 percent of the time you do) does not apply when it comes to gluten and an autoimmune thyroid condition (or any other autoimmune condition as a matter of fact).

Be wary of most soy. It directly suppresses your thyroid function and lowers your metabolic rate. If you don't have thyroid or estrogen issues, you can incorporate a small amount of fermented soy into your diet, but only organic, and not daily—just a few times a week.

Eliminate dairy for a time and then retest to see if your body can handle it. Both the lactose (sugar) and casein (protein) found in most dairy products can be triggers for a runaway inflammatory response in the body. In addition, a recent study showed that when subjects with Hashimoto's restricted lactose, not even 100 percent of the time, their TSH levels normalized. For these reasons, we recommend that our clients (regardless of a thyroid issue) avoid dairy completely during the fourteen-day B3H+ Metabolic Cleanse and the twenty-eight-day Lean Body Phase of the Program. We want to know if they notice a difference in how they feel and look. Many typically lose stubborn fat just by eliminating dairy. After this elimination period, a slow reintroduction of dairy can be made to determine the level of lactose or casein intolerance, although dairy restraint is encouraged if you suffer from any autoimmune condition.

Rebalancing the Thyroid

Because weight gain is often a consequence of thyroid disease, it is critical to tailor your diet to foods that will counteract the negative effects of thyroid dysfunction, support your immune system, and boost overall health.

Here is a sample of our recommended food combination menu for restoring the immune system and thyroid, which will help reignite your fat burning metabolism:

Sample Thyroid-Friendly Menu

Breakfast: _____Lean protein or Protein Packet
                 _____Veggies or low-glycemic fruit
                 (one to two servings per day)
                 _____Healthy fat

Snack: _____Lean protein
(If needed)   _____Healthy fat and veggies

Lunch: _____Lean protein or Protein Packet
                 _____Slow burning carbohydrate* (gluten free)
                 _____Veggies or low-glycemic fruit
                 _____Healthy fat

Dinner: _____Lean protein or Protein Packet
                 _____Slow burning carbohydrate* (gluten free)
                 _____Veggies
                 _____Healthy fat

*Most women who need to lose weight should aim for 50 to 75 grams of net carbohydrates per day. See the Carbohydrate Threshold Chart below. Usually two small starchy servings of carbs per day meet this net carb limit. If the carbs are from green veggies, you'll likely eat more than two small servings per day, as they are higher in fiber and have a lower carb impact. Net carbs are your total grams of carbohydrates minus grams of fiber. See Nutrition Label example below to figure out net carbs in processed foods.

Hormonal Net Carbohydrates:

Goal: <10g Per Serving

(To find Net Carbs: Subtract fiber grams from total carb grams)

NUTRITION LABEL:
Serving Size- .5 cup
Servings Per Container: 4

AMOUNT PER SERVING:
Calories: 90/ Calorie from Fat: 30
Total Fat: 3 grams
Cholesterol: 0 mg
Sodium: 20 mg
Total Carbohydrates: 20 grams
   Dietary Fiber: 5 grams
   Sugar: 11 grams
Protein: 6 grams

The ideal carb limit depends on your unique carb threshold (and your thyroid and adrenal gland health), which does not take into account your activity level, age, current metabolic rate, and genetics.

The following chart will help you decipher where your net carbohydrate threshold is:

Net Carbohydrate Threshold Chart

Based on a 2000kcal Per Day Diet	Percentage of Carbohydrates	Carbs (grams) For Women	Goal and Population
Very low carb	<10%	<50 g	- Neurological issues, Alzheimer's, certain cancers, etc. - Severe blood sugar problems
Low carb	10-15%	50-75 g	- Weight loss - Blood sugar regulation - Mood swings - Digestive Issues
Moderate carb	15-30%	75-150 g	- General health - Maintain weight - Adrenal Fatigue - Hypothyroidism - Familial hypercholesterolemia
High carb	>30%	>150 g	- Athletes and highly active people - Trying to gain weight - Fast metabolism - Pregnant/Breastfeeding

Sample One-Day Thyroid Rebalancing Menu

Breakfast:

- Lean Body Protein Shake

or

- Nitrate- and hormone-free chicken sausage with half a cup mixed berries

or

- Half a cup of "Squirrel Nut Cereal": Mix 2 teaspoons of cocoa nibs, 1 tablespoon unsweetened coconut flakes, ¼ cup unsalted nuts, ½ cup unsweetened almond milk, 1 teaspoon ground flax meal and/or chia seeds

or

- If you're feeling food-prep lazy or just short on time and want to boost your thyroid health, eat a tablespoon of organic unrefined coconut oil. It's a great source of fat and drives your energy levels for hours.

Lunch:

- Protein Packet

or

- Four ounces of grass-fed burger with half an avocado and tomato on a bed of mixed greens with a tablespoon homemade vinaigrette and a teaspoon chia seeds or ground flax meal

or

- Salmon salad swiss chard wraps, plus one serving of fruit

Dinner:

- Protein Packet

or

- Four ounces of rotisserie chicken or grilled mackerel, several cups of colorful veggies, tossed salad with a tablespoon homemade vinaigrette and a teaspoon of chia seeds or ground flax meal with half a small yam or half a cup of wild rice

Snacks:

- Celery with a tablespoon nut butter (not peanut butter)
- Small handful of nuts or seeds with a one-ounce piece of 100 percent dark chocolate
- One low-glycemic fruit (berries, green apples, pears, oranges)
- Raw veggies and half a cup guacamole, hummus, or homemade vinaigrette
- A tablespoon of organic, unrefined coconut oil

Final Words

No two clients are exactly alike, and this is why we personally take a holistic approach to treating our clients with thyroid and hormonal imbalances. When you begin our Balance 3H+ Program, you have access to both a thyroid- and hormone-balancing diet, supplements, herbs, comprehensive testing, and bioidentical hormones. You don't have to go on suffering from the ravages of thyroid disease and perimenopausal and menopausal hormonal imbalances. Your thyroid and hormonally linked mood swings, weight gain, fatigue, cravings, bloating, and other symptoms can be understood and relieved.

We hope this information has been helpful in teaching you more about your thyroid health and how you can begin holistically rebalancing a thyroid condition with proper nutrition and support from knowledgeable professionals. Now that you have read this chapter, you are better equipped to meet with your thyroid specialist to discuss your options and to make lifestyle changes which will be crucial in optimizing your treatment success.

How the B3H+ Program Worked for Me

Name: Mindy

Age: 43

Starting weight: 175 pounds

Total weight lost: 32 pounds

Current weight: 143 pounds

I ate a low-fat diet for over fifteen years and did an hour of cardio nearly every day of the week. No matter what I tried, my weight wouldn't budge from 175 pounds. My energy levels were in the tank regardless of the time of day. When I requested a TSH (thyroid stimulating hormone) test from my primary care doctor, the results came back "normal," which, at a glance, suggested I did not have a thyroid issue. My doctor recommend I try the most popular weight-loss program in the world, Weight Watchers, and also prescribed a conventional weight-loss drug. Within a few days, this drug caused a dangerous drop in my blood pressure and body temperature, in addition to extreme fatigue.

Just as I was about to give up on ever feeling healthy again, I found Dr. Kealy's Balance 3H Plus medical weight-loss program. Dr. Kealy immediately recommended a comprehensive thyroid panel which included T3, T4, reverse T3 and TSH to more accurately diagnose a potential thyroid problem. Although, my T4 and TSH results read normal, my T3 was very low.

The B3H+ healthcare team began treating me and the cause of my hypothyroid symptoms and problems. To correct my sluggish thyroid, I was given a customized T3/ T4 combination therapy treatment. So far, it has been very effective for rebalancing my thyroid hormone levels, and reducing symptoms.

I was also tested for a variety of vitamin and mineral deficiencies. I learned that I was deficient in zinc, manganese, vitamin B12, chromium, and copper. I was given pharmaceutical-grade nutrients and supplements to restore my levels quickly.

I think the biggest physical change for me was my improved energy levels. The Program also included a full metabolic hormone test. My cortisol was particularly high, putting my body in a state of chronic stress and fatigue. The Metabolic Cleanse, Lean Body Shakes, and whole food diet helped reset my hormonal chemistry. Within the first three months of being on the Program, I lost over thirty pounds. Today, I tell all my friends and family members this is a doctor-led medical weight loss and hormonal balancing program with a ton of science behind it. I've got more energy and zest for life today than I did when I was in my twenties, and I lost the stubborn pounds along the way.

References Chapter 8:

1. Amino, N., et al., "Possible Induction of Graves' Disease and Painless Thyroiditis by Gonadotropin-releasing Hormone Analogues," *Thyroid* (2003); 13(8):815–818.
2. Canaris, G. J., N. R. Manowitz, et al., "The Colorado thyroid disease prevalence study," *Archives of Internal Medicine* (2000);160:526–534.
3. Davies, T., et al., "New Genetic Insights from Autoimmune Thyroid Disease," *Journal of Thyroid Research* (2012);2012:6.
4. Leibel, R. L., et al., "Changes in energy expenditure resulting from altered body weight." *New England Journal of Medicine* (1995);332(10):621–628.
5. Mackawy, A. M. H., B. M. Al-ayed, B.M. Al-rashidi, "Vitamin D Deficiency and Its Association with Thyroid Disease," *International Journal of Health Sciences* (2013); 7(3):267–275.

6. Neve, M. J., C. Collins, and P. Morgan, "Dropout, Nonusage Attrition, and Pretreatment Predictors of Nonusage Attrition in a Commercial Web-Based Weight-loss program," Ed. Gunther Eysenbach, *Journal of Medical Internet Research* 12.4 (2010):e69.

7. Roy, A., M. Laszkowska, J. Sundström, et al., "Prevalence of Celiac Disease in Patients with Autoimmune Thyroid Disease: A Meta-Analysis," *Thyroid* (2016); 26:880–890.

8. Shinkov, A., A. M. Borissova, J. Vlahov, et al., "Male Gender Differences in the Thyroid Ultrasound Features, Thyroid Peroxidase Antibodies and Thyroid Hormone Levels: A Large Population-Based Study," *Journal of Endocrinological Investigation* (2014); 37:269.

9. Silverstein, M. G., J. R. Kaplan, et al., "Effect of Soy Isoflavones on Thyroid Hormones in Intact and Ovariectomized Cynomolgus Monkeys (Macaca fascicularis)," *Menopause* (2014); 21(10):1136–1142.

10. Skugor, M., "The Underactive Thyroid: Hypothyroidism" in *The Cleveland Clinic Guide to Thyroid Disorders*. New York: Kaplan Publishing (2009):11–28.

11. Truong, T., D. Baron-Dubourdieu, Y. Rougier, and P. Guénel, "Role of Dietary Iodine and Cruciferous Vegetables in Thyroid Cancer: A Countrywide Case-control Study in New Caledonia," *Cancer Causes & Control* (2010);21(8): 1183–1192.

12. Vojdani, A., and I. Tarash, "Cross-Reaction Between Gliadin and Different Food and Tissue Antigens," *Food and Nutrition Sciences* (2013);(4):20–32.

13. Zimmermann-Belsing T., et al., "Circulating Leptin and Thyroid Dysfunction," *The European Journal of Endocrinology* (2003);149(4):257–271.

CHAPTER 9
FIT AND FIERCE AFTER FORTY

The Balance 3H Plus Reboot Fitness Program

Now that you've learned how nutrition and lifestyle changes can reset your hormones and reawaken your metabolism, it's time to incorporate the final component of our total health program: exercise and movement. In order to maintain your hard-earned weight loss and see new contours in your shape, we want you to couple your new eating patterns and lifestyle practices with our scientifically supported exercise and movement program, appropriately named Reboot. The creator of this cutting-edge exercise program is Lisa Avellino, the B3H+ fitness director and head personal trainer. To learn more about Lisa now, go to www. balance3hplus.com.

Your first several weeks of the Balance 3H+ Metabolic Cleanse and Lean Body program has given your stalled metabolism a jump start, and now your body is at its prime to burn through stubborn fat. Lisa's Reboot program is designed to reignite your fat-burning hormones and regulate your hormonal stress in a positive way.

Why Reboot's Workouts Work

You *really* can achieve and maintain a higher level of fitness and have a toned physique after forty. You might find yourself doubting this statement because it has become much harder to lose the fat than it was ten years ago. Other beautifully seasoned women will agree with you, it does get harder. Fat seems to appear overnight, and weight loss seems impossible to obtain. Plus, there are numerous research studies that support these claims. Unfortunately, women eventually reach their breaking point and resort to another trendy diet coupled with long, arduous exercise in order to painfully lose a few extra pounds. Eventually, frustration grows as willpower fails them again. Complete defeat sets in as there seems little point in suffering for such insignificant drops on the scale.

Over time, the chronic dieting and over exercising leads to a tremendous amount of physical stress on the body. This causes a down regulation of the metabolism leading to greater weight gain, joint problems, emotional issues, accelerated aging. And it puts stress hormones into overdrive exacerbating perimenopausal and menopausal symptoms. These negative side effects and the impact of low-calorie, high-dose moderate to vigorous exercise diets have been well documented in the scientific community. For instance, one study on physical activity and weight control found that high volumes of exercise stimulate hormones like cortisol and others that increase hunger signals (Cook 2011, 419–424). So, if you are running twenty miles a week, you'll lose weight only if you can override the urge to eat additional calories to keep you in energy balance.

Worry no more, the Reboot workouts are exactly what you need in order to further transform your now healthier body into a healthy and fit body after forty. For years, research has supported the power of maintaining hormonal balance and an ideal weight through a slight caloric deficit via diet and exercise that combines elements of both resistance exercise and weight training with circuit training (not long aerobic exercise sessions). This exercise-and-diet formula moves the body toward replacing fat with metabolically active muscle, and helps you avoid weight gain in a healthy way.

Our Reboot personal trainers and fitness coaches will introduce you to a unique approach that involves short bursts of somewhat intense exertion followed by intervals of more gentle exercises and breathing techniques. Unlike traditional exercise programs, our Reboot program enables *you* to control how hard you push during the more intense intervals and how long you spend resting or engaged in more gentle movements. You can pause and rest in the middle of sets or between them. It is totally up to you. By employing the rate of perceived exertion (RPE) scale, *you* determine when you may want to rest and for how long. On the RPE scale, 1 is like lying in bed eating bonbons, and 10 like pushing yourself at your maximum effort and you are struggling to breathe.

Rate of Perceived Exertion (RPE)Scale

1	Resting
2	Really Easy
3	Easy
4	Moderate
5	Challenging
6	Hard
7	Hard
8	Really Hard
9	Really, Really Hard
10	Maximal Effort

With the Reboot program, you are competing with no one but yourself—your previous best. This way you can gauge your intensity on how you feel each day or how you performed during your last workout, not by how hard or how fast someone else is working. Some women take shorter rest breaks—ten to thirty seconds—while others may take fewer rest breaks, but for longer durations.

As you progress, you'll see our Reboot exercise program shift your metabolism to burn fat and sugar, which enhances your results, saves you time, and speeds recovery. It improves lean muscle mass without "bulking" women up to look like bodybuilders. The workouts build strength, aerobic capacity, balance, flexibility, body and breath awareness, and coordination, all which tend to wane with age (especially after age forty) when we don't practice or train.

The Reboot exercise program can be done gradually, so you work your way up to an active lifestyle. We have you start from wherever you are and ask that you commit to self-care and self-improvement by moving and exercising more.

We offer four workout options which fit well into the busiest of schedules. Our fifteen-, thirty-, forty-five-, and sixty-minute workouts condense all of the benefits into one compact, total body session with the right timing, intensity, and rotation of movements to spark a sluggish menopausal metabolism and restore hormonal balance.

Goal of the Reboot Workouts

The goal of all the Reboot workouts is to work synergistically with the B3H+ nutrition recommendations in triggering peak hormonal and muscle responses. With quality nutrients and exercise, along with restorative lifestyle habits, you stimulate feel-good hormones (endorphins) and metabolic hormones (testosterone and human growth hormone), which improve lean muscle mass, decrease inflammation and pain, and offset cortisol production.

Probably one of the most important mechanisms of regular exercise is that, as you stimulate new muscle growth, you also become more sensitive to insulin. This allows fat and carbohydrates to be taken up and metabolized by the working muscles rather than stored in your belly (Poirier 2011, 459–470). This means that, when you eat cake (which should be gluten free and on a rare occasion—right?), your body is better able to deal with the fatty-sugar surges and less likely to store it as belly fat. You also make a lasting change from a metabolism that burns primarily sugar to one that runs on stored fat.

Finally, the workouts are designed to help you continue burning calories from fat for sixteen to forty-eight hours after the workout. This post-workout effect is due to the dramatic changes in hormone levels (for example, increases in testosterone and human growth hormone) that occur during the workout, affecting your body's use of fat and sugar in a positive way after your workout. These workouts also blunt your hunger hormone signals (ghrelin levels), help regulate satiety hormone signals (leptin levels), improve sleep, and increase energy production.

What Is Circuit Training and Why Reboot Uses It

In general, circuit training differs from traditional cardio or aerobic exercises (jogging, walking, biking, or using an elliptical machine) in that it combines elements of cardio exercise and resistance training into one total-body workout. The Reboot circuits alternate brief but intense bursts of activity (both cardio and resistance) that stimulate new muscle growth with less-strenuous active rest types of restorative, gentle movements. The reawakening and growth of new muscle is what signals metabolic hormones to speak directly with your fat cells, liver, and brain to re-engineer your metabolism and hormonal profile. So by circuit training at the right intensity, you'll have more muscle and less fat, which is exactly why the Reboot program uses this training format.

An example Reboot circuit could be a thirty-second sprint (at your current fitness level) on a stationary bike, followed by squats with or without dumbbells for ten repetitions, resistance band overhead shoulder presses, and then a slow but active foam roller massage for the upper and mid-back muscles. This would be repeated two times before moving on to the next circuit of exercises. Note, each circuit typically incorporates into the workouts a slower, more mindful, gentle movement with coordinated breath work similar to what is used in yoga, Pilates, and soft-tissue massage techniques.

When programmed and applied correctly, circuit training produces numerous positive side effects and works with the body's natural healing mechanism. There is so much research on its benefits for anxiety, depression, insomnia, hormones, osteoporosis, obesity, related metabolic diseases, and other conditions (Bemben et al. 2010, 650–656; Martyn-St James et al. 2006, 1225–1240; Loprinzi et al. 2017, 676–685; Morgan 2003, 231–238; Freeman et al. 2007, 230–240). In menopausal women, it's been shown to lower systemic inflammation and stress levels, which directly affects sex, metabolic, and hunger hormones (cortisol, insulin, leptin and ghrelin) (Freeman et al. 2007, 230–240).

Our Reboot workout circuits are quite different from some of the most popular high-impact intensity training (HIIT) programs. Reboot circuits are designed to heal a broken, aging metabolism and reduce inflammation, not create more health problems through exercising too hard or too long. Recent studies suggest that the intensity of the workout matters more, when it comes to fat loss, than the time or type of training (Giannaki et al. 2016, 483–490). Women who do too much continuous exercise at a moderate pace don't lose weight after sticking to this type of exercise program for several months. Our Reboot program won't have you exercising longer; it will have you exercising smarter and *with* your hormones, not against them. The workouts are intentionally speckled with short bursts of intensity in between active, but restorative movements. They work superbly to reset your metabolic hormones to healthy levels.

Reboot Workouts Give You the Power

The type of exercises and the amount of resistance or weights used (if any) will likely be different for everyone. There is also no defined rest period that is always taken between exercises. You control when you rest and for how long. As you become more fit, you'll find that you require less rest and will likely push yourself harder. The exercises in the workouts circuits can be adapted to every age and every level of fitness. For example, one person may do a low-impact march with an alternating strength circuit to protect and reduce force on her joints, while another person may be able to run without any problem.

Another unique feature of our workouts is that they can be done anywhere by using just your body or even things in nature. Be creative! Some of our clients used five-liter water bottles as weights while on vacation in Mexico, and others used logs while running on park trails. Whatever exercise mode and devices you choose to use or not use, it's up to you. But our fitness experts always encourage clients to vary things up every four to six weeks. This prevents stagnation and boredom, lowers injury risk, and keeps it challenging and fun, which is critical to sustaining an active lifestyle. Try changing your training technique by using different workout machines, cable pulley attachments, barbells, dumbbells, grip variations, or resistance bands. Get out on your bike, run or walk the bleachers at your local high school, use the community around you to create your own workout playground.

The Reboot Exercise Programs

Reboot 15

This fifteen-minute workout is designed to help you get used to the unique total-body exercise program, to ensure that you have correct form while performing exercises, and that you progress slowly into the program to avoid injury or creating unnecessary soreness. For some of you, fifteen minutes of exercise may seem overwhelming. We get that. But you've got to start moving more. So no matter how little you've done up till now, commit to moving just five minutes a day. Take a brisk walk, jog up the stairs at work, or march in place. Just find some way to move even a little bit. At the end of each week, add another five minutes until you are moving for fifteen minutes straight through. Then, come back and use your newfound confidence and stamina to begin the Reboot 15.

The Reboot 15 Workout Rules:

1. Do this circuit training workout every day for fifteen minutes, for at least two weeks.
2. Complete a two- to five-minute dynamic warmup by doing one round of the same exercises in the circuit, but slowly, and through a full range of motion.
3. Do each exercise ten times and immediately start the next.
4. Do each circuit, repeating each exercise with control and mindfulness for two rounds before moving onto the next.

5.   Use the rate of perceived exertion (RPE) scale in this chapter or a heart rate monitor to determine your level of work intensity at any given time. Remember, you get to tailor your workout to your individual fitness level. Rest when you need to, and then start again where you left off.

6.   Stretch and incorporate calming breathing techniques for at least five minutes to cool down and recover.

7.   These fifteen-minute workouts emphasize the quality of movements performed, not the number of repetitions or how fast. We want you to practice combining the exercise principles with mindful movements and coordinated breathing while you work out.

The Reboot 15 workout sample looks like this:

Circuit 1:
1.   Pelvic tilt—supine
2.   Leg extension quadruped
3.   Cat-camel
4.   Breathing

Circuit 2:
1.   Bridge—double and single leg
2.   Side-lying clam
3.   Shoulder clocks
4.   Half front plank—knees

Circuit 3:
1.   Bilateral external rotation
2.   Brugger postural relief position
3.   Wall slides—scapula retraction

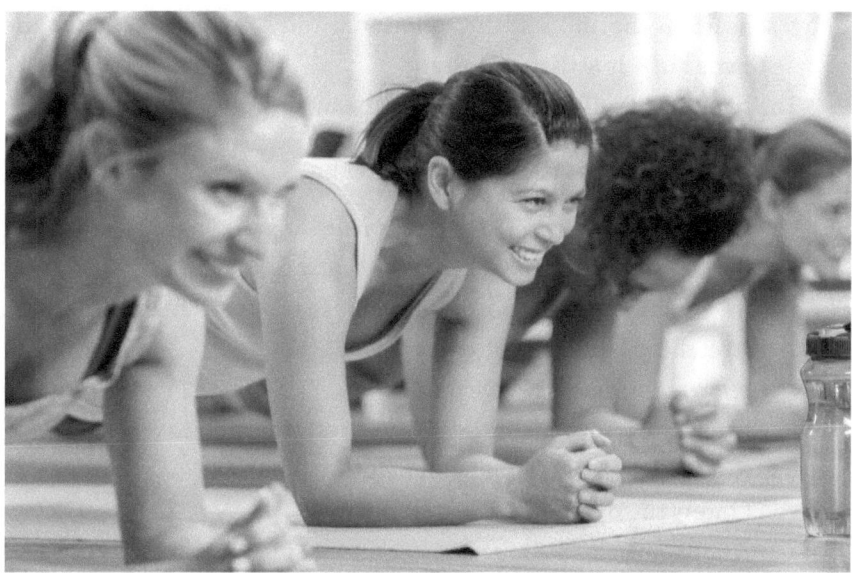

Reboot 30

This thirty-minute workout is more advanced and slightly harder than the fifteen-minute workout because it incorporates self-myofascial massage techniques into the circuits. *Myo* means "muscle," and *fascial* relates to the "band" or "connective soft tissue" that surrounds the muscles, nerves, bones, and organs of the body. Self-myofascial massage is a simple self-treatment method for your soft tissues (muscles, ligaments, tendons, fascia, and skin), nervous system (sensory nerve endings), and blood vessels that helps your body continue to run smoothly and efficiently and makes it less apt to develop aches and pains in the first place. It gives you the ability to treat yourself and interrupt the downward spiral of stress and dysfunction that, over time, stores itself in your body and can cause pain. It can improve posture, help you recover from exercise, improve movement performance, and ultimately improve the integrity of your all tissues. The self-myofascial release techniques will help you stay healthy, youthful, and active for a lifetime. As a critical component of the Reboot program, it will change your understanding and relationship with your body, sensations, hormones, and emotions, and it may also change the course of your life. It is that important!

The benefits of self-myofascial massage include:

- Increases in local blood circulation
- Rehydrates the area (known as profusion)
- Releases knotted masses of tissue and adhesions
- Makes corrections and connections in tissues that daily exercise, stretching, and yoga often bypass
- Helps minimize scar tissue
- Improves joint capsule health and restores mobility
- Lowers stress hormones and emotional holding
- Quiets the nervous system
- Aligns muscles with bones so that you move with efficiency and ease
- Teaches you how to develop a new relationship with your body, and how to support your body's natural healing mechanisms, in addition to unlocking the specific points of pain and "stuck stress."

We also encourage you to perform other types of restorative exercise that work synergistically with the Reboot workouts, such as daily, long restorative walks, tai chi, yoga, and qi gong.

The Reboot 30 Workout Rules:

1. Do this circuit training workout *every other* day, for thirty minutes each day. In addition, you should walk every day for at least thirty to sixty minutes. We suggest walking a minimum of thirty minutes on the days you do your Reboot workouts and longer on off days. Walking works synergistically with the Reboot workouts in helping regulate your hormonal stress response in a positive way.

2. After a two- to five-minute dynamic warm up without added resistance, do each exercise ten times and then immediately start the next.

3. Optional: add body weight resistance during workout, although, this should only be done when appropriate in the circuit and if you have beautiful form performing the movements with no resistance.

4. Do each circuit, repeating each exercise for two rounds, before moving on to the next circuit.

5. Rest only when you need to. Use the rate of perceived exertion (RPE) scale in this chapter or a heart rate monitor to determine your level of work intensity at a given time. Also, pay attention to body sensations that can tell you when you are working hard enough. They include: sweat, breathlessness, slight burning sensations in the muscles, or general fatigue. These are all indicators that you may need to rest. But they are also signs that you are creating a metabolic shift into fat burning mode.

6. Stretch and use myofascial methods, and incorporate calming breathing techniques for at least five minutes to cool down and recover.

The Reboot 30 workout sample looks like this:

Circuit 1:
1. Pelvic tilt—supine
2. Leg extension—quadrupled
3. Cat-camel
4. 4-square breathing
5. Arm-leg raise (aka deadbug)

Circuit 2:
1. Bridge with tubing
2. Side-lying clam
3. Hamstring curls on stability ball
4. Foam roller thoracic mobility
5. Shoulder clocks

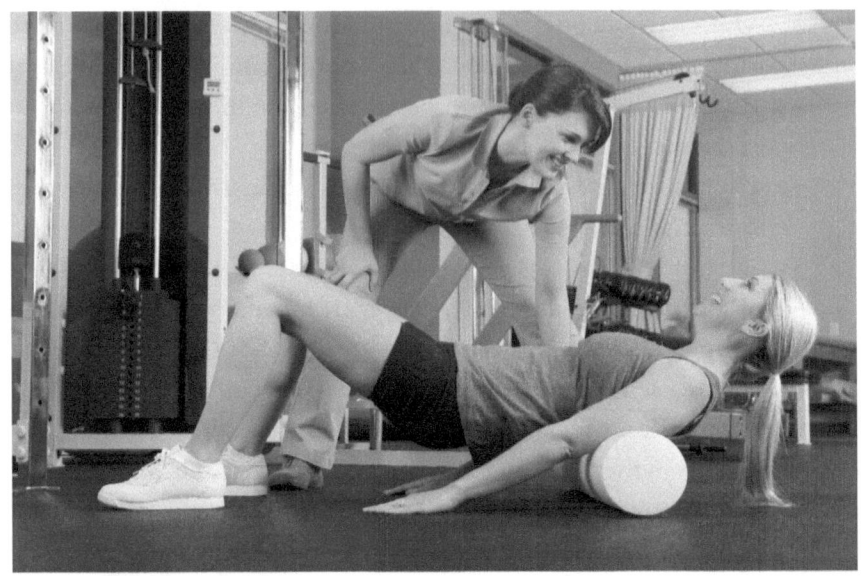

Circuit 3:

1. Bilateral external rotation
2. Brugger postural relief position
3. Wall slides—scapula retraction
4. Standing hip abduction

Circuit 4:

1. Wall push-ups
2. Scapula retraction—protraction
3. Wall sit isometric hold
4. Abdominal bracing

Circuit 5:

1. Side plank
2. Stability ball transfers
3. One-leg standing
4. Foam roller adductors

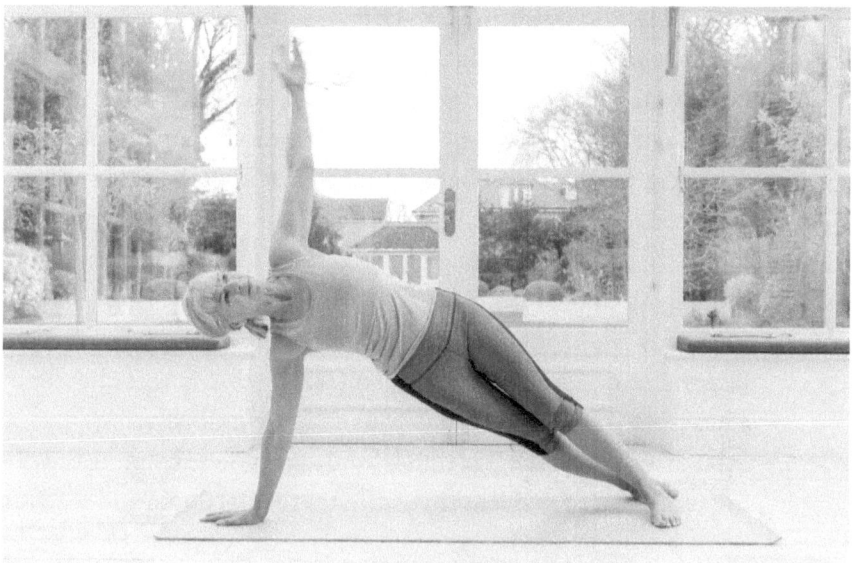

Reboot 45

This Reboot 45-minute workout involves short periods—less than one minute—of more intense exertion followed by one to two minutes of active recovery or moving at a lower intensity that allows you to catch your breath and your heart rate to recover. It is specifically designed to boost your metabolic hormones, such as human growth hormone and testosterone, which aids in building and maintaining muscle, counteracts the negative effects of the stress hormones, and supports fat burning.

The Reboot 45 Workout Rules:

1. Do this circuit training workout three to four days a week for forty-five minutes each day and watch yourself get leaner, stronger, and more energetic. In addition, keep walking every day, accumulating to at least thirty to sixty minutes, walking longer on your off days.

2. After a two- to five-minute dynamic warm-up without added re-
    sistance, do each exercise ten times and immediately start the
    next. Add resistance here to make the exercises are more chal-
    lenging. Focus on using resistance bands or light-to-moderate
    free weights, like dumbbells, sandbags, or kettlebells to increase
    the intensity.
3. Do each circuit, repeating each exercise for two rounds before
    moving on to the next circuit.
4. Rest only when you need to, then start again where you left off.
    Use the rate of perceived exertion (RPE) scale in this chapter or
    a heart rate monitor to gauge your exercise intensity.
5. Stretch, use myofascial methods, and incorporate calming breath-
    ing techniques for at least five minutes to cool down and recover.

The Reboot 45 workout sample looks like this:

Circuit 1:
1. Cat-camel
2. Cross crawl quadruped
3. Breathing
4. Bridge—tubing

Circuit 2:
1. Side-lying clam
2. Bilateral external rotation
3. Foam roller thoracic mobility
4. Standing hip abduction
5. Shoulder clocks

Circuit 3:
1. Wall sit
2. Knee push-ups
3. Seated rows
4. Hamstring curls— supine

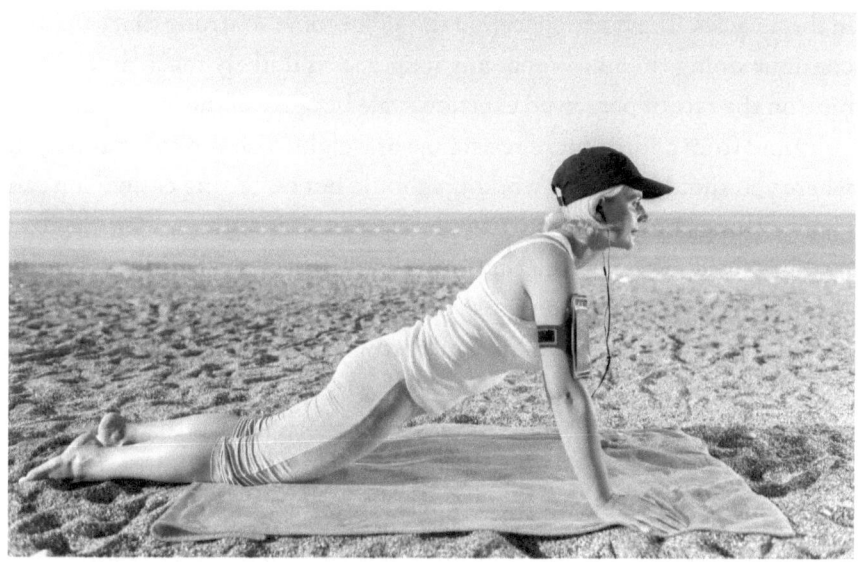

Circuit 4:

1. One-leg standing
2. Shoulder horizontal abs standing
3. Abdominal bracing arm and leg raise
4. Shoulder extension

Circuit 5:

1. Foam roller adductor
2. Wall slide—arm elevation
3. Plank—feet wide—lateral
4. Psoas roll

Reboot 60

This Reboot 60-minute workout has similar positive effects as the Reboot 45 workout on your metabolic hormones and in making you stronger, firmer, and leaner. The major difference in the Reboot 60 is you begin increasing the resistance (the amount of weight lifted) in the workouts and add advanced exercise techniques designed to generate an intense "burn" in the muscles. The burning feeling should become so strong that you can't continue doing the movement any longer. You'll likely reach an eight or nine on the rate of perceived exertion scale because of the increased difficulty and from adding more resistance or weight. This is perfect and right where you should be. Your workouts should not be getting easier. You can change things up by adding new exercises each month, lighten the load by 20 percent, but increase the work time slightly, or the pace in which you move through the exercises. You can also add power exercises like burpees, jump squats, medicine ball throws, squat thrust, or box jumps.

You'll also be giving yourself more time to rest in this workout. Start by giving yourself one to two minutes recovery in between sets that are difficult and more strenuous. Although you don't want to completely recover, so only take enough rest to allow you to continue. This will be different for everyone. Some of you may need only a minute, and others may need the full two minutes or more. As you get stronger and more fit, you will likely require less rest between sets. You want to strive to keep your muscles working hard throughout the whole exercise set. But you absolutely need breaks so you can push yourself hard again when you move on to the next challenging exercise. When done safely and with beautiful, correct form, the value of these workouts is priceless. You'll become stronger, boost your metabolism, and greatly increase the time it takes to lose weight without creating hormonal havoc in the body.

The Reboot 60 workout rules are the same as the Reboot 45 workout rules.

The Reboot 60 workout sample looks like this:

Circuit 1:
1. Cat-camel
2. Cross crawl—quadruped
3. Bridge—tubing
4. Side-lying clam

Circuit 2:
1. Bilateral external rotation
2. Foam roller thoracic mobility

3. Standing hip adduction
4. Foam roller squat using band

Circuit 3:
1. Knee push-ups
2. Step-up
3. Squat, hold, 'n' row
4. Shoulder extension

Circuit 4:
1. Ab bracing arm-leg
2. Foam roller adductor
3. Wall slide—arm elevation
4. Elbow or hand plank on toes

Circuit 5:
1. Psoas roll
2. Half side bridge
3. Shoulder retraction
4. Reverse fly

Knowing When the Reboot Workouts Are Working

Within a week of starting our easy-to-follow Reboot workouts, you'll notice a redistribution or loss of water weight. Many fat-storing hormones indirectly influence how the body carries water weight. You (and others) will notice your face and abdomen are thinner or more defined. The waistband of your pants will feel looser by a half an inch to an inch. You will experience five to ten pounds of additional weight loss, which may come from water weight but is also a good indicator that you are moving into burning fat more efficiently. As you shift into burning fat, you'll notice the shape of your buttocks, hips, fat above the knees, and upper arms will become noticeably leaner and more toned. You'll feel lighter, you'll have greater motivation to work out, and you'll have more endurance and energy. The Reboot workouts will become easier, you'll feel less muscle soreness, and you'll recover quicker.

How the B3H+ Reboot Program Worked for Me

Name: Leslie

Age: 41

Starting weight: 205 pounds

Total weight lost: 29 pounds

Current weight: 176 pounds

I tried every diet and exercise in the universe, but never lost weight. I had a low, lean-muscle-to-body-fat ratio, poor endurance and strength, but had incredible flexibility and loved to walk. Being more advanced in a few areas but so "behind" and challenged in others was preventing me from losing the weight and looking and feeling my best. I needed to create a healthy total-body exercise practice without over straining myself or just going through the motions. The Reboot circuits had me working muscles I had neglected for years. It kept me motivated because it was fun, challenging, but achievable. I felt and saw changes within a brief period of time. After I followed the Reboot exercise program for three months, my cardiovascular stamina and strength improved dramatically. I now enjoy lifting weights and the short burst of somewhat uncomfortable intensity that is inserted into the workouts. The best part is that I broke through my weight loss plateau. My body-fat percentage dropped by several percentage points, and I lost nearly thirty pounds.

The B3H Plus Reboot Program Core Principles

You *can* stick to your new exercise and movement program! Use these secrets from the creator of the Reboot exercise program, Lisa Avellino, to help you stay (or get back on!) track.

1. **Monitor personal accountability and attitude.** To develop a plan of accountability, surround yourself with supportive, motivating, positive people who will help you get to the next level. At B3H+ centers, we are your critical-care support team. We guide you every step of the way to keep you from running out of steam, and we will celebrate with you when you bust through a plateau. We also make accountability easier because we teach you exercises and restorative techniques that balance your hormones, speed up your metabolism, and get you to your weight loss goal.

2. **Rely on the pleasure principle.** Ask yourself what activities you enjoy, and then incorporate them into your exercise routine. We want you to get inspired to stick with this for life. We want you to get hooked on exercise and healthy, restorative movement. When you engage in activities that you enjoy, you'll not only reach your health goals, but you'll notice positive changes in your mood, outlook on life, and even in the world around you. Exercise does not have to feel like an arduous task. Our creative, fun, and challenging Reboot program will help you discover a whole new world of feeling energized, capable, and fit. You'll turn into one of those people who feels "off" when they go too many days without the joy of exercise.

3. **Put your emotions in motion.** Are you feeling blue? Has hormonal havoc got you down or feeling crazy? Are you tired, feeling "hangry" (hungry + angry), unmotivated, or overwhelmed? The quickest way to change your emotional state is to get moving. Even a small amount of physical activity, like walking a few flights

of stairs, offers you an immediate mood boost. It works quickly every time. It costs nothing, and it doesn't harm you in any way. It only relieves toxic thoughts and feelings. Try a quick Reboot fifteen-minute stress relief session and a cup of hot decaffeinated green tea.

4. **Don't skip your end-of-workout cool down!** The cool down is definitely the most under-appreciated aspect of an exercise program. But, in Lisa's expert opinion, at the top in importance for health and hormone balance. Try walking for fifteen minutes, gently stretching, and doing myofascial release to relieve tension from a particularly grueling workout. Cool down gives the body a chance to return to a state of rest, repair, and recovery. It allows you to slow everything down after you've pushed yourself and amped up your nervous system. Aim effortlessly to restore your normal stress-free breath cycle. A normal, natural breath cycle starts with a deep inhale through the nose which allows the abdomen and ribs to expand vertically and horizontally. This is followed by a complete exhale out through the nose. You'll also want your pulse rate under a hundred beats per minute by the end of your training session.

5. **Get to bed earlier**! Aim for a bedtime around ten o'clock. Make sure your room is dark like a cave and cool. Inappropriate sleep—either too much or not enough—will silently sabotage your exercise performance, weight loss goals, and hormonal balance. Research has also shown that avoiding artificial light, TV, and other electronic screen activity several hours before going to bed improves sleep (Smolensky et al. 2015, 1029–1048).

6. **Create daily "me time."** This is when you listen to music, meditate, breathe deeply, or gently massage yourself. Whatever you do, just be in the present moment and make it calming. Release all your anxiety, anger, and stress. Visualize these emotions leaving

every area of your body. Negative thought patterns are insidious and difficult to release. Over time, they can hijack your heart, mind, and body without you ever realizing it. This is why "me time" is the best time to detoxify your mind. Give yourself a few worry-free minutes of "me time" every day. You deserve it!

7. **Stay hydrated!** We've said this before and will say it again because it is super important that you remain hydrated to stay healthy. Drink water throughout the day and sip during your workouts. If you are not getting enough water, it will be difficult to reach your fat-loss and fitness goals. It is a super nutrient and also a valuable tool for controlling hunger and appetite before and between meals. One study had participants drink large glasses of water an hour before meals. Doing so significantly blunted their hunger and reduced their caloric intake at the meal (Davy et al. 2008, 1239–1239). Water is one of your greatest allies in achieving the complete benefits from the Balance 3H+ program. As with everything else, how much water you should drink depends on your individual makeup and activity level. Listen to your body and drink the right amount for you. To guarantee adequate hydration, drink enough water so that your urine is consistently light yellow or almost clear in color.

8. **Seek variety.** If you walk outdoors on the same path every day, attempt to notice one thing that's different on the path—an emerging flower, the smell of the air, changing of the leaves, the sunlight and clouds—or take a different route each time. Connecting with Mother Nature stimulates the mind and nourishes and calms the body and soul. The B3H+ Reboot workout is by no means an equivalent to Mother Nature, but it does offer you similar benefits in that it provides a variety of stimulating and nourishing movement patterns. The exercises, combined with the elements of mind, body, and breath awareness, add to the restorative, hormone-balancing effects. The workouts engage all your senses and create a natural state of well-being.

9. **Find a workout partner.** Exercising with a friend has been shown to increase effectiveness in all wellness programs (Grave et al. 2011, 11). The B3H+ program is one of your new workout partners. We are here for you with new workout and exercise ideas, expert trainer advice, and motivational tips. Plus, we offer a variety of easy ways to incorporate our fast and fun Reboot total body workouts into the busiest of days.

10. **Keep your eye on the prize.** If you are running out of steam, and still have weight to lose, you can throw in some of these plateau busters:

    - Double-up your workouts. Try a long walk in the morning and a late afternoon resistance training session, or vice versa.
    - Increase the intensity of your workouts by adding a bit of resistance or going lighter and for more repetitions. You can also add a variety of different styles of training to create more burning or temporary fatigue in your muscles; for example, jump squats or stationary bike sprints.
    - Try a B3H Plus metabolism-boosting supplement and replace two meals a day with the B3H+ Lean Body Functional Food shakes.
    - Drink more green tea to help boost your metabolic rate.
    - Get hot in the sauna after a workout to increase the release of muscle building, fat-burning hormones.

11. **Write it down.** Finally, define your health and weight loss goals and objectives in a journal. Map out your personalized exercise program, logging all your sets, repetitions, and resistance. You are not alone. We are here to guide you in the process of reinvigorating your life and setting you on track for a brighter tomorrow.

12. **Treat yourself.** Most diet and lifestyle programs focus only on what you need to avoid or take out in order to achieve your weight

loss goals and stay in shape. At B3H+ we want you to go out and give yourself rewards that match the big and small, seemingly insignificant achievements that you have and will continue to accomplish. Now when we say rewards, we don't mean food rewards. We want you to start focusing on building in a weekly and monthly non-food reward system that keeps you happy with your new body and motivated to continue this healthy new way of eating, moving, and being. Here are some of our favorite reward ideas: a massage, a manicure or pedicure, a facial, new exercise clothing, a bubble bath with essential oils, a new book, a pair of walking or training shoes, or time out for peace in a place you enjoy.

Final Words

Here at B3H+, we want to communicate the message that movement is very much like medicine. Knowing *what* type and intensity of movement to practice, and *when* you need to rebalance and heal yourself is similar to knowing what type of herb or medicine you need when you are recovering from an illness. Certain types of exercise, like the Reboot circuits, combined with other healthy, restorative movement and breathing practices, can address very specific perimenopausal and menopausal issues and symptoms.

Remember, if you are new to exercise always start with the basics, with Reboot 15 and daily walks. Then, after several weeks, move to our higher-intensity and more challenging circuits with (or without) added resistance or advanced exercise variations in the Reboot 30, 45, and 60 workouts. The key is to progress slowly. It takes time to shift your physiology into fat-burning mode and rebalance your hormones. But, with the adjustments you've already made in diet and lifestyle, you'll achieve faster results from the Reboot exercise program. You'll see dramatic changes in your physique. You'll be motivated to continue your workouts. You'll feel more athletic and look forward to doing other physical activities like biking, hiking, and swimming with friends and family. You'll have reached a happy state of awareness about your body that you've never experienced before. You'll have an innate understanding about what it takes for *you* to become and stay lean, hormonally balanced, healthy, and fit for life!

How the B3H+ - Reboot Program Worked for Me
Name: Sylvia
Age: 54
Starting weight: 115 pounds
Starting body fat %: 29 percent
Ending body fat %: 21 percent
Current weight: 117 pounds

At five four, I weighed 115 pounds, and all my friends and family would comment at how trim I was. I wore expensive clothes that flattered my small frame, but I did not like what I saw in the mirror when I was naked. I had no muscular definition in my legs, arms, or abdominal wall, and was shaped like a banana—straight up and down. When I began the Reboot program, I measured in at 29 percent body fat. To my surprise, I fell into the overweight, at-high-risk-for-metabolic disease category. Boy, was I shocked! Lisa, B3H+'s fitness director and personal trainer, did an amazing job in explaining that, even though I was five pounds underweight and thin in appearance, I had a higher ratio of fat to muscle, which was why my body fat percentage registered high. After eight weeks on the Reboot and B3H+ Program, my percentage decreased to 21 percent. I gained several pounds of metabolically active muscle, and am now seeing definition and curves where I want them. Lisa taught me that muscle is denser than fat, which is why my weight did not change, but it also takes up less space, so I look more lean and fit. My mindset about health and body size has changed for the better. I no longer worry about just losing weight, but about increasing and maintaining lean muscle mass in order to keep my body fat at a healthier percentage.

How the B3H+ - Reboot Program Worked for Me
Name: Gena
Age: 51
Starting weight: 176 pounds
Total weight lost: 12 pounds
Current weight: 164 pounds

I was suffering from night sweats, sleeplessness, and prolonged stress, which all were contributing to my menopausal mood swings, weight gain, and fatigue. Lisa's Reboot circuits and restorative self-care practices helped me lower my cortisol levels. I was stunned with the weight loss, which was not the primary reason for starting my journey to better health. My sleep improved, I felt calmer, and I had more energy. I felt at peace with myself. The gains I made in the program are ones that are sustainable and have taught me how to care for my mind, body and spirit.

References Chapter 9:

1. Bemben, D. A., et al., "Effects of Combined Whole-body Vibration and Resistance Training on Muscular Strength and Bone Metabolism in Postmenopausal Women," *Bone* (2010)47:650–656.
2. Cook, C. M., and D. A. Schoeller, "Physical Activity and Weight Control: Conflicting Findings," *Current Opinions in Clinical Nutrition and Metabolic Care* (2011)14:419–424.
3. Davy, B. M., et al. "Water Consumption Reduces Energy Intake at a Breakfast Meal in Obese Older Adults," *Journal* of the *American Dietetic Association* (2008)108 (7):1239–1239.

4.   Freeman, E. W., et al., "Symptoms Associated with Menopausal Transition and Reproductive Hormones in Midlife Women," *Obstetrics & Gynecology* (2007) Aug;110(2 Pt 1):230–240.

5.   Giannaki, C. D., et al., "Eight Weeks of a Combination of High Intensity Interval Training and Conventional Training Reduce Visceral Adiposity and Improve Physical Fitness: A Group-based Intervention," *Journal of Sports Medicine and Physical Fitness* (2016) 56(4):483–90.

6.   Grave, Riccardo Dalle, et al., "Cognitive-Behavioral Strategies to Increase the Adherence to Exercise in the Management of Obesity," *Journal of Obesity* (2011) 2011:11.

7.   Loprinzi, Paul D., et al. "Cross-sectional Association of Exercise, Strengthening Activities, and Cardiorespiratory Fitness on Generalized Anxiety, Panic and Depressive Symptoms," *Postgraduate Medicine* (2017) 129:7:676–685.

8.   Martyn-St James, M., and S. Carroll, "High-intensity Resistance Training and Postmenopausal Bone Loss: A Meta-analysis," *Osteoporosis International* (2006) 17:1225–1240.

9.   Morgan, K., "Daytime Activity and Risk Factors for Late-life Insomnia," *Journal of Sleep Research* (2003) 12:231–238.

10. Poirier, P., and J. P. Despres, "Exercise and Weight Management of Obesity," Cardiology Clinics (2011) 19:459–470.

11. Smolensky, Michael H., Linda L. Sackett-Lundeen, Francesco Portaluppi, "Nocturnal Light Pollution and Underexposure to Daytime Sunlight: Complementary Mechanisms of Circadian Disruption and Related Diseases," *Chronobiology International* (2015) 32:8:1029–1048.

CHAPTER 10
THE BALANCE 3H PLUS PROGRAM FOR LIFE

While working with our clients, I've noticed that those on the B3H+ program meet weight-loss goals and see results faster than those on calorie-counting diets. I've also seen those clients have long-term continual success in making powerful bodily transformations. A hormonal approach to fat loss provides so much more than weight loss. For instance, hormones in balance will positively affect moods and emotions. The connection between hormones and mental health is well documented, and if you are a female who has gone through puberty, perimenopause, or menopause, you know this from first-hand experience. When your hormones are stable, so, too, are the mood swings; but this works in reverse too. When your mindset is more positive, every cell in your body is impacted. When you feel good about yourself, you're more motivated to adhere to a healthy lifestyle.

Your outlook on your life, health, and wellness goals are channels for hormonal changes that profoundly affect your body. For instance, if you are feeling sad, staying motivated and focused on the program can be difficult. You may end up falling prey to your old habits of seeking out certain comfort foods or eating too much to avoid feelings of sadness. Feelings of happiness and satisfaction with your body and life lead to greater motivation to continue with the Program. Thus, you must bring your mind, body, and emotions into balance with each other in order to sustain the full transition into hormonal harmony. Take a daily mental inventory or journal about the things in your life that make you feel balanced and centered. What are they? Do feel better about yourself because of your practice of eating whole foods and natural detoxification? Are supportive supplements helping? What about periodically slowing down your pace of life and lowering stress so you can eventually "move faster" but while feeling better? Are you setting aside time each week for things you love and enjoy? All of these help you experience a greater sense balance.

Visualization is another way you can rebalance your mind and emotions. Envision yourself harnessing the power to change any automatic negative thoughts, beliefs, and behaviors that hold you back from total health and being the person you are meant to be. Look internally at the things that make you feel imbalanced. Identify each, close your eyes, and visualize them as individual sailboats on the open sea. They may be your greatest challenges, unconscious but long-held beliefs about yourself or others, your incessant worries, old habits, or behaviors that draw you away from the health and body you desire. Imagine each sailboat traveling further and further from the forefront of your mind's eye, becoming so small that eventually all you see is a speck of a boat in the distance. You are letting them sail away, one by one. As you imagine this, let your unconscious mind experience and sense whatever comes up from inside you. Maybe it's a sense of weightlessness, vibrancy, openness, relief, compassion, healing, sadness, or fear of letting go of something so familiar to you. This is an example of a visualization practice that opens space for change and for restoring balance. It also is a tactic for gaining a greater connection with your purpose for changing, focus, and choice. Every single time you engage in this type of practice, you set into motion signals that imprint these images in your brain as your new reality, as if it were really happening. The more you do this, the more effective it will become and the more improvements you can create in your everyday life. This new way of being and thinking releases you from the oppression of the old ways.

Your ultimate formula for long-term change must include a strong, intimately connected *why* or purpose for seeking and sustaining good health, the right amount of focus, and the continuation of healthy choices that sustain hormonal balance and fat loss. There are two things we immediately do with our new clients. First, we uncover the underlying hormonal imbalances that are holding their health and fat-burning capacity hostage. As you have learned, this is not an easy task. Secondly, our health experts address the emotional aspects of long-held, limiting-beliefs and negative self-talk that impact their capability to sustain change. This can be the most difficult to overcome. At times, we all can find ourselves challenged by limiting beliefs and deleterious self-talk. But we cannot let these or other perceived challenges derail us from our paths of knowing that our purpose, focus, and habits, over time, will bring about the results we desire. By taking the information and tools you have learned in the Program, you can quickly reconnect your choices to the bigger and more meaningful present moment. You can tap into your true *why*—your driving force—to stay ultra focused in pursuit of your desires. Here and now is the moment in which your health future lies. Your power of sustaining hormonal change and balance is at the level of the mind and spirit as well as the physical body.

So go ahead, right now, and write down your purpose for changing—your *why*! Make it so important that you'd be willing to risk your life for it. This way, you'll put the highest price you could pay on having good health if you quit or rest on your laurels. Maybe you're changing for your children, or maybe it's a personal scare with a disease. Whatever your *why* is, write it down and read it often so you never forget your innermost reason for pursuing a better body and life.

Next, continue to focus on practicing the small, seemingly insignificant daily nutrition and lifestyle habits that you've developed here in the Program. The rewards will not always come in the form of pounds lost and may not appear obvious at times, but they can be easier to recognize if you live in the moment. Find gratitude for how much you've grown, and honor yourself for the extraordinary efforts you've put into your B3H+ Program. Trust that your commitments to your new diet and lifestyle will continue to pay off in terms of fat loss, physique changes, and in living younger longer. Notice your new taste buds that are now hungry for nutrient-dense foods, not sweet treats or heavy breads. Notice how well your body moves and feels now that you've been doing the Reboot workouts and managing your stress. Notice that your hormone issues have vastly improved (or have even dissolved) and that you have a steady flow of natural energy and are sleeping restfully. This metabolic balance will keep you happy and glowing with better health and motivated to sustain your new self-care, self-loving practices for the rest of your life.

Sustenance!

Maintaining the B3H+ Benefits

You now hold all the necessary tools required to attain a well-balanced, vibrant, healthy body: a nutritious and balanced diet; periodic detoxing; consistent and varied types of exercise and restorative mind-body-spirit practices; a balance of work and leisure; sufficient sleep; and love and support from friends, family members, and health role models and experts. These are all meant to help you remain focused on your purpose and reach your goals. Once you've hit your ideal number on the scale or are at a point where you feel completely balanced again, you may think you've reached the end of your health journey. However, the hardest and most critical phase is before you—the maintenance phase! This is considered the hardest because of the grim statistics of how most diet and lifestyle changes fail over time. But, because you approached your health and weight loss from a hormonal versus a calorie-only perspective, you are already ahead of most at making new habits stick. We know from working with hundreds of women over the years that the real work of maintenance begins when the B3H+ eight-week program comes to an end. Maintenance is never about reaching a destination point; rather, it is a dynamic process that continues well after the pounds have dropped.

The gateway to maintaining healthy weight and hormonal balance is about making everyday choices (the small and big) that either bring you closer to or further away from living longer, leaner, healthier, and happier.

One of the first things you need to do when you notice yourself slipping back into old self-defeating habits (eating and drinking too much, walking and working out less, not sleeping, not journaling, not managing stress, and so forth) is to enact a plan with specific actions for what to focus on according to where things are going wrong. This plan will keeps you moving in the right direction. Here is our guide for resetting your fat-burning hormones and restoring balance in your body. These actions steps will get you back on track as quickly as possible so you can maintain the B3H+ Program benefits for life!

1. Surround yourself with support. Find others who have established healthy habits and will support the changes you are making rather than sabotaging you. There is a saying we love and strongly believe in: You are the sum of the five people you spend the most time around. In other words, you become who you hang out with the most. If you want to get better at anything, you'll likely naturally gravitate toward people who already have what you want—a dream job, a great physique, and knowledge or mastery of a skill or subject—eating for their metabolism or diet, for example!

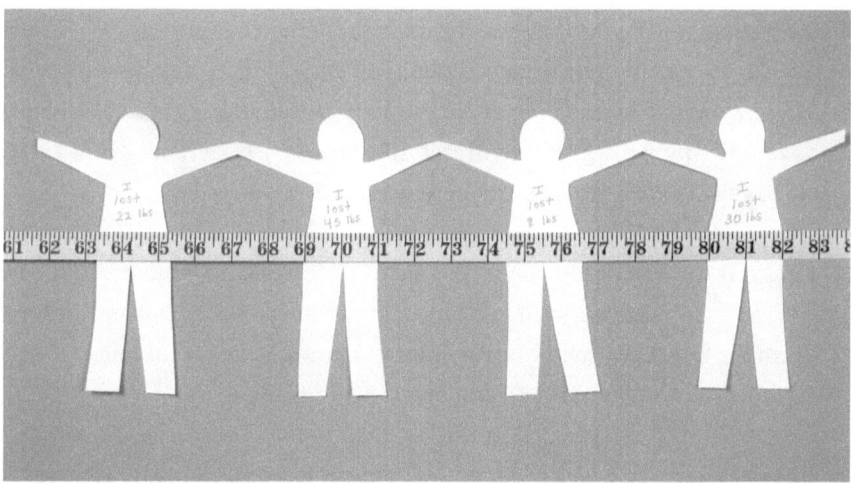

2. Make it real—write it out. If you get to a plateau or feel stuck, you'll want to go back to journaling your food information, including your level of hunger, your mood, your energy, and your cravings; scheduling your exercise times; tracking your hours of sleep; and recording other health-promoting habits. This enables you to identify where you need to tighten things up. For instance, you notice you are overeating and experiencing hormonal cravings lately, so you start tracking your health parameters again and see that you've been skimping on your sleep to watch late-night TV. Because you've completed the B3H+ Program, you already know that, if you get to bed earlier, you can reset your hunger hormones and prevent weight gain. When you write it out, you can zero in on things and track your progress and see regressions. A writing habit ensures a continuous hormonal accountability and enables you to make adjustments and take charge of your choices.

3. Dial in your diet. Ask yourself, are you eating enough protein and healthy fats? Aim for 20 to 30 grams of protein per meal and incorporate a healthy fat source on every plate of food you eat. Are you limiting refined carbohydrates? In our experience, our most successful fat losers keep their refined carbohydrates to a minimum, and their total net carbohydrates between 50 and 75 grams per day depending on activity levels, thyroid health, and cortisol (stress) levels. (Revisit Chapter 8, Rebalancing a Low Functioning Thyroid, to review the carbohydrate threshold chart.) More active days typically allow for a higher carbohydrate intake; however, on less active days, you need fewer carbs. To maintain your optimal weight, choose slow-digesting carbohydrates, like veggies, 99 percent of the time. Eat a large salad or a pot of veggies at least twice a day.

4. Shake it up. We recommend you go back to making your B3H+ Lean Body meal replacement drinks for breakfast and lunch (or dinner). Remember how they help diminish cravings and quickly fill you up with satiating, hormone-balancing pea protein and fiber.

5. Get greened. To quickly get yourself moving forward again with lightness and more clarity, shift your body's pH from acid to alkaline by drinking your greens. This boosts metabolism, helps remove estrogen-disrupting chemicals, improves thyroid function, and rids the body of extra toxins that may be circulating. Try a warm cup of homemade pH-balancing broth before breakfast and then later in the day for a little pick-me-up. It's the perfect way to get your detoxifying greens!

6. Fill with fiber. Include lots of raw and slightly steamed veggies and add fiber-rich foods like chia and ground flax seeds, not only to fill you up, but to sweep out that toxic residue. Make sure you are pooping like a champ at least once per day.

7. Slip in more sleep. Recent studies show that getting adequate sleep (seven to nine hours) each night is critical to maintaining and improving insulin sensitivity, preventing you from developing insulin resistance and, subsequently, type 2 diabetes (Broussard et al. 2016, e40–e41). When you don't get enough sleep, specifically hours of REM (rapid eye movement) sleep, you become prone to storing more of your calories as excess body fat. Allow your sleep to be an easy and quick hormone reset for you.

8. Watch less, move more. Maintain a consistent level and variety of exercise modes, and minimize daily screen time. Research suggests that people who maintain their weight loss over a ten-year period of time average less than ten hours a week in screen time (Helajärvi et al. 2014, e101860).

9. Cultivate positive emotions and relax deeply. Intentionally choose a low-stress life by cultivating a mind-body-spirit restoring practice. This is an essential part of maintaining health and internal peacefulness. People who consciously work at cultivating positive thoughts (and some days you'll have to work at this more than others), emotions, intentions, and beliefs directly affect their body's ability to heal, relax, and be well (Sakallaris et al. 2015, 40–45). They also have an easier time recognizing and transforming negative psychological states like depression, anger, and anxiety (Garland et al. 2010, 849–864). Return to a restorative movement-breathing practice, like our Reboot 15, or make time for a gentle yoga or meditation session. We also recommend a hot Epsom salt bath with your favorite essential oil added. Create a relaxing mood by lighting the bathroom with candles and resting your head and back on a soft bath pillow. Take slow, steady deep breaths and pamper yourself often.

10. Reduce, remove, rebalance, repeat. This strategy is employed by most of our clients who have been successful at attaining and maintaining their optimal body changes over the long term. Don't wait until you've gained ten pounds of body fat to take action. Reduce and then remove all sugar-fatty foods, drinks, and other products that are not serving your goals and can make you feel sluggish, heavy, hungry, out of control, and reliant on willpower. Replace your reliance on willpower by shifting your diet and exercise habits when your hunger, emotions, cravings, and energy are getting the best of you. This rebalances your hormones. Then, repeat the B3H+ Program every three to six months to keep your metabolic hormones in check, eliminating the need for will-fail willpower.

11. Take your B3H+ supplements. Our high-quality, pharmaceutical-grade nutritional supplements can help sensitize your cells to insulin, lower cortisol, detoxify, nourish, and rehab the body. Supplements help you get to the next levels in rebalancing your metabolic hormones. See a list of all our products and nutraceutical supplement line at https:// balance3hplus.com

12. **Test, don't guess.** At B3H+ we have a "science first" approach for every component of the Program, providing success to our clients in sustainable leanness and total health. Testing yourself is a perfect and scientifically valid way to measure and track your progress. How? There are many valid and reliable ways to test your weight loss progress and health maintenance outside of using a typical scale, which tells you nothing about your body composition or hormonal balance. The following are handy self-tests to measure and track your progress:

a. Learn how to perform an at-home fasting blood sugar (glucose) test each morning before you exercise, eat, or drink anything. And do several two-hour-postprandial (after meal) tests for three days, recording your results. You want to fall within the "optimal" values for fasting blood sugar, not just within the "normal" values of 65 to 99 mg/dL. Levels too close to the cut-off can be damaging to body tissues (heart, brain, blood vessels) and increase risk for numerous diseases (Garber et al. 2008, 933–946). Anything below 90 mg/dL for fasting blood sugar is your goal and indicates you are at a low risk for developing diabetes and cardiovascular disease. Postprandial blood sugar levels should drop below 120 mg/dL within two hours after a meal according to the most current scientific literature (Tirosh 2006, 87-88; Nichols et al. 2008, 519–524; Garber et al. 2008, 933–946). Something to note: the medical establishment's definition of "normal" is more common than optimal and isn't a good guide for the results you desire.

Periodically testing your blood sugar gives you important feedback on how quickly your body is removing sugar from your blood, indicating your cells' receptors are sensitive to insulin's call to take up sugar. This simple self-test can also give you insight to how your body uniquely reacts to different glucose-rising foods (such as quinoa as opposed to sweet potatoes) that may or may not cause negative effects. Finally, self-glucose monitoring may also help protect you from developing insulin resistance, prediabetes or other complications. Keep in mind that you should not to rely on a single blood sugar marker. Healthy people can still have postmeal blood sugar spikes above 140 mg/dL. Please consult an integrative physician if you are interested in learning more about glycemic control or have concerns with your blood sugar patterns.

b. Invest in a body-fat scale. This simple device lets you know how much fat versus muscle you are losing, which enables you to be completely aware during your transformation. Once you have made your transformation, we suggest you use this to track your progress and check your body-fat percentage. This will reinforce you in maintaining your ideal set body-fat percent level. Use your scale to check your percentage once a week at the same time in the morning, before you work out or eat or drink anything. If one morning you measure yourself and you are up a few percentages, that's an all-out warning sign that it's time to refocus and get back to the program basics which keep you on the B3H+ path.

c. To monitor your nightly sleeping heart rate, breathing patterns, and REM cycles, we like the OURA Ring Sleep tracker for unbeatable accuracy. Other devices that work well for tracking sleep cycles and understanding your quality of rest are the Fitbit Blaze or Charge 2 models.

d. Track your hunger, cravings, mood, and energy signals between meals and snacks. These symptoms are scientific clues to how your body is functioning hour to hour, day to day. Tuning into the clues your body is sending, such as fatigue when you are hungry, cravings when you don't sleep, or lingering soreness after workouts, offers powerful and reliable information regarding your metabolic processes and hormonal balance.

Quantitatively, you may not be able to test these body signals, but they are still reliable expressions that can aid you when it comes to metabolic balance and burning fat. Listen to your body when you receive these powerful signs and make the appropriate adjustments based on your unique biological makeup. For instance, if you're hungry and having cravings, get to bed earlier and eat slightly more protein and tons of fibrous veggies that day. Plus, avoid all refined carbohydrates until you are feeling back in balance.

e. Test your heart rate. This gives you valuable information about how your body is responding to the foods you are consuming. Perform the following steps:

- Before you eat a food that you typically avoid because you know it leads to inflammation, hunger, blood sugar dysregulation, gut issues, and so forth, take a seated heart rate for ten seconds. Multiple that number by six to get your resting heart rate.
- Next, eat a meal or food that you've historically reacted poorly to eating.
- Wait ten minutes and check your heart rate again. If it's gone up by more than ten beats per minute, this suggests you're experiencing a food sensitivity reaction. Thus, you'll either want to avoid eating that food again or limit it to the rarest of occasions and expect some negative reactions to occur. Typically, and depending on the food and your unique biology, reactions may include digestive

distress, joint aches, excess mucus production, itchy skin, and rashes. Please note that some reactions may linger or be delayed three to four days.

f. Heart rate monitors (HR) or the rate of perceived exertion (RPE) scale (in chapter 9, Fit and Fierce After Forty) are great ways to tailor your workouts, assess your intensity and recovery, measure your progress, and stay motivated to train. Remember, the highest proportion of fat is burned primarily after you work out. The amount of fat burned is influenced greatly by the intensity of the workout, not the length. Our Reboot workouts are designed with this in mind. They consist of short bursts of somewhat hard, intense work that spike your heart rate. The bursts are followed by longer, slow, more restorative movements that allow your heart rate to fall again. The real fat-burning hormonal response occurs because the body is pushed hard for a very brief period, near your estimated 80 to 85 percent heart-rate maximum (age-predicted using HR monitors). HR monitors and RPE scales both monitor exercise intensity. If you chose to get feedback from a HR monitor, you'll want to know these age-predicted heart rate equations:

$$HR_{max} = [\text{women: } 206 - \{0.88(\text{age})\}]$$
$$HR_{max =} [\text{men: } 208 - \{0.7(\text{age})\}]$$

Next, take 85% of age-predicted HR_{max}

$$HR_{max} \times .85 = 85\% \text{ of } HR_{max}$$

Example: Let's say you're a forty-year-old women:

$$206 - \{0.88(40)\} = 171 \text{ HRmax (beats per min—BPM)}$$
$$171 \times .85 = 145 \text{ BPM}$$

145 BPM is 85% of the age-predicted HRmax, and is the target HR for this forty-year-old woman while engaged in vigorous activity.

Final Words

You are now ready for a wonderful healing journey to begin—or continue! Although I guarantee you'll notice the weight loss, I hope you realize that the B3H+ program is about so much more. It's about helping you gain mastery over your life, health, and well-being. When you feel hormonally balanced, youthful, sexy, confident, in touch with your body, and at peace in your mind, amazing things can happen. When you adhere to the B3H+ principles outlined in this book, you'll soon feel and look healthier than you do today. Every meal, every workout, and every choice you make to take care of yourself saves you from misery in menopause, years of yo-yo dieting, premature aging, and ill-health. Thousands of women trust our team of integrative health and medical experts to help them live their happiest, most connected and balanced life.

I welcome you to join them!

References Chapter 10:

1. Broussard, J. L., et al., "Two Nights of Recovery Sleep Reverses the Effects of Short-Term Sleep Restriction on Diabetes Risk," *Diabetes Care* (2016);39(3): e40–e41.
2. Garber, A., Y. Handelsman, et al., "Diagnosis and Management of Prediabetes in the Continuum of Hyperglycemia—When do the Risks of Diabetes Begin? A Consensus Statement from the American College of Endocrinology and the American Association of Clinical Endocrinologists," *Endocrine Practice* (2008); 14(7):933–946.
3. Garland, E. L., et al., "Upward Spirals of Positive Emotions Counter Downward Spirals of Negativity: Insights from the Broaden-and-Build Theory and Affective Neuroscience on The Treatment of Emotion Dysfunctions and Deficits in Psychopathology," *Clinical Psychology Review* (2010); 30(7):849–864.
4. Helajärvi, H., et al., "Exploring Causality between TV Viewing and Weight Change in Young and Middle-Aged Adults. The Cardiovascular Risk in Young Finns Study," Ed. Robert L. Newton, (2014); *PLOS ONE* 9(7):e101860.
5. Nichols, G. A., et al., "Normal Fasting Plasma Glucose and Risk of Type 2 Diabetes Diagnosis," *The American Journal of Medicine* (2008);99(6):519–524.

6. Sakallaris, B. R., et al., "Optimal Healing Environments," *Global Advances in Health and Medicine* (2015);4(3):40–45.

7. Tirosh, A., "Normal Fasting Plasma Glucose Levels and Type 2 Diabetes in Young Men," *New England Journal of Medicine* (2006); 354:87-88.

APPENDIX

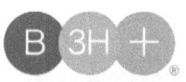 MY WEEKLY GROCERY LIST
SHOPPING DAY_____

POULTRY – Organic, Free-Range, 97% Lean	QUANTITY
○ Chicken Breast (skinless, white meat)	4 oz
○ Turkey Breast (skinless, white meat)	4 oz
○ Applegate Turkey Bacon	4 slices
○ Applegate Turkey, Chicken, or Ham Cold Cuts (plain)	4 oz

MEAT – Organic, 97% Lean	QUANTITY
○ Grass Fed Beef	4 oz
○ Pork loin or tenderloin	4 oz

EGGS – Organic, Free-Range	QUANTITY
○ Egg whites	6 oz

SHELLFISH – Organic, Wild Caught	QUANTITY
○ Clams	4 ½ oz
○ Crab	4 oz
○ Lobster	4 oz
○ Mussels	4 ½ oz
○ Oyster	4 ½ oz
○ Scallops	4 oz
○ Shrimp	4 oz

FISH – Organic, Wild Caught	QUANTITY
○ Anchovies (fresh, canned in water)	4 oz
○ Cod	4 oz
○ Flounder	4 oz
○ Halibut	4 oz
○ Mackerel	3 oz
○ Mahi Mahi	4 oz
○ Octopus	4 oz
○ Salmon	4 oz
○ Sardines (fresh, canned in water)	4 oz
○ Sea Bass	4 oz
○ Snapper	4 oz
○ Sole	4 oz

FISH – Organic, Wild Caught	QUANTITY
○ Squid	4 oz
○ Swordfish	4 oz
○ Tilapia	4 oz
○ Trout	4 oz
○ Tuna (fresh, canned in water)	4 oz

HEALTHY FATS	QUANTITY
Avocado	1/4 or 1 sm
Raw Unsalted Nuts (except peanuts)	1 oz
Oils (olive, coconut, grape, any seed oil)	1 tb
Olives	4-5

VEGETABLE – Organic	QUANTITY
○ Acorn Squash	½ cup
○ Alfalfa Sprouts	½ cup
○ Artichoke (fresh, canned in water)	1 cup
○ Arugula	1 cup
○ Asparagus	1 cup
○ Bok Choy	1 cup
○ Broccoli	1 cup
○ Broccoli Raab	1 cup
○ Brussels Sprouts	1 cup
○ Butternut Squash	½ cup
○ Cabbage	½ cup
○ Carrots	½ cup
○ Cauliflower	½ cup
○ Celery	1 cup
○ Collard Greens	1 cup
○ Cucumber	1 cup
○ Eggplant	½ cup
○ Escarole	1 cup
○ Jicama	1 cup
○ Kale	1 cup
○ Lettuce (all)	1 cup
○ Mushrooms	½ cup
○ Okra	½ cup

VEGETABLE – Organic	QUANTITY
○ Onion	½ cup
○ Peppers (all)	½ cup
○ Pickles	½ cup
○ Snap/Snow Peas	1 cup
○ Spaghetti Squash	½ cup
○ Spinach	1 cup
○ String Beans	1 cup
○ Swiss Chard	1 cup
○ Tomato	½ cup
○ Yellow Squash	½ cup
○ Zucchini	½ cup

FRUIT — ORGANIC	QUANTITY
○ Apple	1 small
○ Blackberries	½ cup
○ Blueberries	½ cup
○ Clementine	½ cup
○ Grapefruit** (check with interaction with meds)	5 ½ oz
○ Kiwi	½ cup
○ Nectarine	½ cup
○ Peach	½ cup
○ Pear	½ cup
○ Plum	½ cup
○ Pomegranate	2 oz
○ Raspberries	½ cup
○ Strawberries	½ cup

STARCH — ORGANIC	QUANTITY
○ Mary's Gone Crackers	5 crackers
○ Paleo Bread: Almond or Coconut	1 slice
○ Scandinavian Bran Crispbreads	2 crispbreads
○ Suzie's Whole Grain Brown Rice THIN cakes	4 cakes
○ Sweet Potato	½ cup

Balance3hplus.com

ABOUT THE AUTHOR

Mitchell R. Suss prides himself on maximizing the health and lives of menopausal women through his company's proprietary breakthrough metabolic weight loss program, Balance 3H Plus. Over the past twenty years, he has helped thousands of women look, feel, and live life younger. Suss currently lives in Hartsdale, New York.

www.ingramcontent.com/pod-product-compliance
Lightning Source LLC
Chambersburg PA
CBHW030441290526
45786CB00001B/388